Treating Troubled Adolescents

TREATING TROUBLED ADOLESCENTS

A Family Therapy Approach

H. Charles Fishman

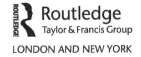

Routledge
Taylor & Francis Group

LONDON AND NEW YORK

First published 1988 by Hutchinson Education Ltd.

This edition published 2015 by Routledge
27 Church Road, Hove, East Sussex, BN3 2FA
711 Third Avenue, New York, NY 10017

First issued in paperback 2015

Routledge is an imprint of the Taylor & Francis Group, an informa business

ISBN 13: 978-1-138-87201-1 (pbk)
ISBN 13: 978-0-09-182279-8 (hbk)

To My Family

CONTENTS

FOREWORD

OR THE FIRST HALF of this century our concept of adolescent problems pertained to inner hydraulics in disarray, or to social upheaval generated within a context of peers. Therapy for disturbed adolescents focused on individual dynamics or group treatment, and, for the most part, did not take into serious consideration adolescents in relation to their families. Adolescent problems were regarded as due mostly to the internal difficulties inherent to the stage of life, and the family was seen mainly as a backdrop to the vicissitudes of personal development. To this day, even among family therapists, such a view colors our understanding and limits our ability to help troubled adolescents.

This excellent book, by one of family therapy's most creative practitioners, changes all that. Exclusively devoted to elaborating a family-therapy model of understanding and treating adolescents, it is a major contribution to the field. It also performs the unique and much-needed function of revitalizing the concept of homeostasis, moving it from its status as a general explanation for non-change to that of a useful principle for organizing therapeutic dialogue.

With exceptional clarity and sensitivity, Charles Fishman shows where and how homeostasis operates in families and how recognizing and working with each family's "homeostatic maintainer" can produce significant change. In addition to clarifying the concept of homeostasis, the book provides a carefully articulated set of assessment tools. But it does much more than that. It effectively translates theory into workable clinical interventions. The cases presented here—on runaways, suicide, incest, violence, and other serious problems that affect adolescents and their families—vividly dramatize how a few well-grounded ideas can powerfully enhance therapeutic encounters.

Any clinician who has been ready to give up in frustration when dealing with the thorny problems of adolescent patients will welcome this thoughtful, practical book. It promises to sharpen the lens of every therapist both inside and outside family therapy.

—BRAULIO MONTALVO

ACKNOWLEDGMENTS

I HAIL FROM CHICAGO. Carl Sandberg's "city of big shoulders" was, as I remember it, a very practical, no-nonsense industrial city. Although extremely beautiful, Chicago had little patience for frivolity. My hope is that this book will have a kind of impatient, Midwestern practicality—useful to the practicing clinician who needs to work, and at times work fast, to address difficult situations. I should be very satisfied if this volume served as a useful companion for such a clinician, who is every day confronted with severely troubled adolescents and their families.

I have centered the book on severe difficulties that adolescents are confronted with. Of course, there are many other problems that come to therapy, and my hope is that the clinician will be able to extrapolate from the cases in this book to those many other problems.

Through serendipity I seem to have found myself at the right place at the right time. During the last fifteen years, I have been so extremely fortunate as to be in a position to work with and learn from very wise people. As a young therapist, I was supervised by Jay Haley and Salvador Minuchin. I then had the invaluable experience of writing the book *Family Therapy Techniques* with Dr. Minuchin. Carl Whitaker and I did a number of workshops together, an important learning experience for me. Influential colleagues who contributed to my views of therapy are: Virginia Goldner, Brad Keeney, Jamshed Morenas, and Olaf Ulwan.

In some of the cases in the book I was a consultant to either a trainee or a colleague. I would like to acknowledge Cecile Herscovici, William Johnson, Cheryl Jones, Bill Mathews, and Olaf Ulwan for their erstwhile efforts in helping these families change. I also want to thank Judith Landau Stanton for her creative supervision of one case in the later stages of therapy.

This volume might not have seen the light of day were it not for the tireless efforts of Sheila Doyle, who transcribed, corrected, and expertly helped edit the case transcripts. I want to acknowledge Sheila for her tireless attention to the innumerable details which must be attended to if a volume such as this is ever to be published.

Braulio Montalvo, my friend and mentor, was an inspiration during the time that it took to complete the book. I want to add to the long list of book acknowledgments that consistently credit him as the most brilliant and helpful midwife of nascent ideas in the field. For this book, however, Braulio was more than just a beacon of conceptual clarity. He provided the necessary encouragement and precious friendship.

Another person who was instrumental to these pages' seeing the light of day was Steven Edelheit. He gave me invaluable editorial assistance, turning my writing into writing. Similarly priceless was Nina Gunzenhauser, who did the fine editing, rendering logic to my loose associations.

Finally, I should like to thank my family: Anu, my sixteen-year-old resident consulting expert on adolescence; Zev, who teaches me daily the wonders of development; and my wife Tana, who read, suggested, read more—and created a context of loving support and encouragement.

PART I

THE THERAPEUTIC

APPROACH

1

Family Therapy: The Treatment of Choice for Adolescents

> O chestnut tree, great rooted blossomer,
> Are you the leaf, the blossom or the bole?
> O body swayed to music, O brightening glance,
> How can we know the dancer from the dance?
> —WILLIAM BUTLER YEATS

A S YEATS (1928) suggests, to think of a part as separate from the whole, of an active subject like a dancer independent of the dance, is absurd. Treating the troubled adolescent apart from an ongoing social context is equally absurd. And yet there are therapies that do just that—treat the troubled adolescent in isolation or solely in terms of a developmental stage subject to a variety of predictable problems.

Of course there is a pediatric, or purely biological, view of adolescence: just as frogs evolve from tadpoles, so do human adults develop from adolescents. This is unarguably true, and no doubt there are physical changes that have very real psychological consequences. But this view does not take us far in trying either to understand or to treat the problems associated with troubled adolescents. We need something more. It is my contention that adolescence must be looked at as a social, rather than a biological, transformation and that this psychosocial approach is the only useful way of conceptualizing the problems and advancing the possibilities for effective treatment.

"Adolescence," then, does not exist apart from a defined social context. To appreciate this fact, we need only to consider that a hundred years ago our grandparents neither conceived of nor experienced adolescence as we do today. As Michael Rutter argues, the very idea of adolescence is a creation of the psychosocial forces at work at a given time.

> Adolescence is recognized and treated as a distinct stage of development because the coincidence of extended education and early sexual maturation have meant a prolonged phase of physical maturity associated with economic and psychosocial dependence; because many of the widely held psychological theories specify that adolescence *should* be different; because commercial interests demanded a youth culture; and because schools and colleges have ensured that large numbers of young people are kept together in an age-segregated social group (Rutter 1980).

Philippe Aries (1962) further contends that the current phenomenon of adolescence arose after World War I. At that time, he argues, young soldiers began to perceive themselves as a distinct and exploited class and subsequently longed to retain their distinction and rebelliousness as a form of protected self-differentiation, a way of distancing themselves from the older generation in control.

Thus "adolescence" has come into existence to fill a need. It is a creation of social forces at work in our culture and cannot be considered apart from its social context. Therefore, it follows that our treatment of the problems associated with adolescence must also take into consideration the social context. In other words, what is needed here is a contextual therapy. Without such a therapy we risk falling into the trap Gregory Bateson (1979) noted in his "dormitive principle": we expend our energies treating the *name* of the problem rather than the context that creates and maintains it. As therapists treating adolescents, we should not be in the business of treating the name of the difficulty—delinquency, suicidal behavior, anorexia, and so on. Instead we should be focusing our attention on the social context that is creating and maintaining the problem at hand.

Why Family Therapy?

The most powerful social therapeutic intervention for working with adolescents is family therapy. Out of the multifaceted context impinging on the adolescent—family, peers, school, idols, culture—the ecologically oriented therapist starts with the pivotal point, which is the family. The family is the social environment out of which the adolescent emerged. It is the source of the most enduring relationships and the adolescent's primary financial support. And the family frequently has the most resources with which to make changes.

Of all the social systems impinging on the adolescent, changes in the family have the most effect on the youngster. These changes include those within individual family members, such as midlife crisis, illness, and career decisions, as well as changes in family development, like children leaving home, divorce, and parents approaching retirement. The adolescent is extremely vulnerable to such contemporary changes within the family structure.

The existence of a disturbed adolescent in a family serves as the silent canary does in a mine—it is a tipoff that there are problems in the system. In addition to being strongly affected by the family context, adolescents in turn affect the context of which they are a part. The very presence of a troubled adolescent in the family creates pressures that require the therapist to pay attention to the other family members. It is only ethical that the therapist address the problems of the context as a whole. Not to do so—to treat just the adolescent in isolation—is to fail the other family members.

What is the Power of Family Therapy?

Family therapy is an approach that transforms dysfunctional interactional patterns between significant individuals and social forces in a person's life. There are a number of reasons why this approach is particularly powerful. First, the family therapy model allows the clinician to see causation as circular as well as, at times, linear. This means that, rather than focusing always on a chain of cause and effect, the therapist has the flexibility to look at the system as a self-reinforcing circle—in some cases a vicious cycle—or as a self-feeding chain reaction. Let us take as an example a case we will explore further in the chapter on violence. In this circular system, the father comes home drunk and fights with the mother. Not surprisingly, the mother and children talk about the man behind his back and are very cold toward him. The father then feels so bad about being treated this way that he goes out and drinks, and the whole circular reaction begins again.

In some cases the therapist can deem a sequence linear and intervene appropriately—for example, by telling parents, "The two of you, by always bailing your son out of jail, are allowing him to stay a delinquent."

The power of circular causation is that the therapist can enter any part of the system, work with as many parts of the system as are available, and eventually transform the entire system. In our example of the violent family, obviously it is not enough to treat just the adolescent who is having problems because of the father's violence. By entering the system, the therapist can disrupt the circular pattern and begin to effect change for all family members.

The family therapy approach is further distinguished by its emphasis on including all significant people and attempting to work with all of the contemporary social forces that are maintaining behavior. Unlike therapies that deal with troubled relationships in a person's life by role-playing and discussions between strangers or by discussion of the problems individually with the therapist, the focus is always on real people with whom the adolescent has difficulties as well as on a search for options to ameliorate those difficulties.

Another characteristic that makes the family therapy model so powerful is that it deals with contemporary social patterns that the therapist actually sees in operation. The great advantage here is that the therapist can work with these patterns, observe change, and gauge the success of the therapy as it goes along.

Lastly, the power of the family therapy model derives from the central notion of the multifaceted self. This is a positive, optimistic approach that regards each individual as having functional facets that can be expressed if the context changes. Thus the problem resides not in the individual but in the context, and by changing the context, different, more functional behaviors can be allowed expression. This approach is very different from diagnostic therapies which look for "illness" embedded in the individual and often confirm the self-fulfilling negative expectation that many such therapy models encourage. Family therapy believes in the perfectability of people—it believes in selves that, to paraphrase Walt Whitman, are large and contain multitudes. By transforming the context, the family therapist seeks to bring forth the best from that multitude, to enhance social interactions, and to allow people to function as capably as possible.

Why is Family Therapy Effective?

How effective is the family therapy model in treating troubled adolescents? A considerable amount of research has demonstrated it to be effective indeed. One study of anorexic children by Salvador Minuchin, Bernice Rosman, and Lester Baker (1978) found that within two to seven years follow-up, 86 percent of the adolescent patients not only were symptom free but were functioning well in terms of their psychosocial status. Additional studies have demonstrated that compared to other forms of treatment, family therapy is equal or superior in effectiveness (Goldenberg and Goldenberg 1985).

There are a number of specific reasons why family therapy is so effective. In the first place, characteristically it leads to the rapid amelioration of problems. For example, the cases cited in this book, in which I was the primary therapist, had an overall treatment course that lasted from four to nine months. The treatment of such severe problems by other therapy models generally would have required a much longer period of time. Now, I am suggesting not that my particular therapeutic approach is unique, but rather that the model itself is especially effective. Many studies have confirmed that family therapy is a brief therapy that leads to a more rapid amelioration of symptomatology than do other treatments, such as psychoanalysis or individual therapy (Bruch 1973).

Another reason why family therapy has proven so effective is that it involves all of the significant people in the life of the adolescent. This inclusiveness means that changes tend to be maintained, because the family system itself, not just individuals, is being transformed. In other words, since all family members undergo change, their mutual changes tend to reinforce and maintain one another. In other therapies the therapist may successfully work with a patient and help bring about the emergence of greater self-awareness or functional self-expression. But often the patient then goes home only to be reprogrammed to follow the old rules of the system and to find the old counterproductive patterns re-emerging. With family therapy, however, all members are a part of the transformation, so the chances for maintaining new, more productive behaviors are much greater.

Family therapy is also more effective because it actively respects the family members by including them in the treatment process. It sees the family not as an external encumbrance that is likely to disrupt therapy, not as a necessary evil, but instead as a resource to facilitate healing. The very idea of family therapy implies confidence in the family as a place for healing. This is a radically different notion from that which informs most other therapies—that a child goes to an expert to be "fixed" because the family has failed and, once fixed, will return home somehow distanced from the old, bad family context.

One last point about the effectiveness of family therapy: it costs less. Because the course of treatment is shorter, because all family members receive treatment but are not billed individually, and because the recidivism rate is much lower, the family therapy approach is less expensive and a more productive use of resources (Lieberman 1987).

Who Are Our Patients?

Before going on, it is important to understand just what we mean by the "troubled adolescent" population. What we do *not* mean is that *all* adolescents, as a group, are prone to serious developmental problems. However, one should keep in mind that the popular understanding of adolescence is that it is a time of deep emotional difficulty. Indeed, the psychoanalytic view has long supported this idea, seeming to regard adolescence as a period of psychosis with everyone in the appropriate age group a potential patient. "The teens are emotionally unstable and pathic," G. Stanley Hall (1904) remarks in an early work. "It is a natural impulse to experience hot and perfervid psychic states characterized by emotion." Later psychoanalytic literature continued to support the idea of adolescence as a normal period of emotional instability and disequilibration (Blos 1979).

But the latest studies contradict the notion that *Sturm und Drang* is a normal, necessary part of adolescence. Indeed, Daniel and Judith Offer (1975) found that only 20 to 30 percent of the adolescent population experience severe difficulties, and that psychic storm and stress are not at all the norm. As the Offers say, those adolescents who are in the midst of severe identity crises and turmoil are not just experiencing a normal part of growing up. What they are experiencing is abnormal, and they are in need of help. The Offers' conclusions have been supported by the work of researchers such as Michael Rutter (1980) and Stella Chess and Alexander Thomas (1984), who have done large-sample, longitudinal studies that confirm that normal adolescents are not necessarily pathic. Our patients, then, are that 20 to 30 percent of adolescents who are experiencing severe developmental problems.

What Are the Issues that Respond to Family Therapy?

This book is based on the premise that adolescents dealing with severe developmental problems respond best to a family therapy approach. There are a number of common issues that surface frequently in our patients and that need to be discussed briefly here.

IDENTITY

The quest for identity is central to the very experience of adolescence, and identity issues often represent a major area of conflict. How do we understand "identity"? Erik Erikson (1958) defined it as some central perspective and direction that each youth must forge for him or herself, "some working unity, out of the effective remnants of his childhood and the hopes of his anticipated adulthood." This view seems to presuppose that the adolescent grows up in a vacuum. But the view of family therapists in general is that not only is the adolescent struggling for identity, the other members of the family are also changing. And it is within this family context that the search for identity gets played out.

There are many possible scenarios within the family context that might provoke an identity "crisis." Is there a disabled sibling, for example, drawing off the family's emotional resources and leaving the adolescent unconfirmed? Is the child struggling for identity in a social situation in which there is a paucity of role models—for example, a family with no adult females? These are the kinds of problematic identity situations that a contextual therapist can best address, by working to create a context within the family that will nurture the transformation from child to adult, pulling together, as Erikson put it, all of those effective remnants and hopes. Family therapy offers a more complete system of therapeutic intervention. Meeting individually with an adolescent struggling with identity issues would be valuable only to the extent that the therapist might provide a substitute role model while helping the adolescent to find someone in his/her socialized environment.

The family therapy approach to issues of identity is supported by research that suggests that adolescent maturity is gained within the context of progressive and mutual definition of the parent-child relationship, with the emphasis for the adolescent placed on maintaining rather than leaving the relationship (Grotevant and Cooper 1985). The family therapist looks at actual interactions and seeks to enhance the process of identity formation by encouraging negotiation between generations. It is this process of negotiation that builds a sense of self in the adolescent; it is a process of confirming mutual respect.

In contrast to traditional conceptions of adolescence as a time for breaking the parent-child bond, family therapy seeks to bring about a gradual renegotiation of the bond "from the asymmetrical authority of early and middle childhood toward, potentially, a peer-like mutuality in adulthood" (Grotevant and Cooper 1985). To achieve identity, Erikson (1968) says, adolescents must forge for themselves some central perspective and direction. Family therapy places its emphasis on a process of forging *with* and *together*. After all, the goal for the family is not to have the child *run* away from home, but to *walk* away from home, and in so doing maintain an appropriately supportive relationship for both generations.

SOCIAL COMPETENCE

The development of social competence is another essential task during adolescence. As Steven Brion-Meisels and Robert Selman (1984) have pointed out, this involves the "construction of new strategies for dealing with changes in interpersonal relationships and for redefining the adolescent's sense of self in the light of new societal and social realities." What better place is there for constructing such strategies and redefining one's self-image than the family. After all, the family is a laboratory for learning social skills; as such, it should become a primary resource for the therapist in addressing difficulties the adolescent may have in this area.

Family therapy can enhance social competence by transforming the adolescent's indwelling social rules of interaction. These rules are formed and maintained by the family and tend to be generalized to external situations. A good example of this extension of family rules to nonfamily social situations is the case of the adolescent who has difficulty in dealing both with siblings and with peers. In situations such as this, the problem can result from the siblings not being on an equal footing with one another within the family. There may be a coalition between one parent and one of the siblings that causes the troubled adolescent to feel incapable of successfully negotiating stable, fair, and flexible relations. The child in coalition who operates from a position of perceived power may refuse to negotiate with peers altogether, while the child subject to the coalition may feel powerless, so may not learn negotiation skills because they are seen as useless. In either case, the result is a problem in socialization in which the adolescent fails to operate competently with peers. By working within the family to redefine the indwelling social rules, the therapist can help the troubled adolescent reform his or her social self into one that is better able to approach both peers and outside power figures such as teachers or employers.

The power of family therapy to address patterns of social interaction works not only from the family outward to the world, but also the other way around. Family therapy can intervene in the adolescent's external social environment—school, peers, community, job—to correct dysfunctional patterns that in turn affect the family. Looking at the real-world context as it affects the adolescent's social development can lead to some surprising insights. For example, the common wisdom is that employment enhances social competence in adolescents. This may be true in many cases, but recent research has found that it does not apply to all situations. Although work may improve personal responsibility and self-management, it does not necessarily build social responsibility, especially where adolescent boys are concerned. In fact, according to research by Lawrence Steinberg and associates (1982), employment may lead to diminished involvement in school, family, and peer commitments, to the development of cynical attitudes toward work, and to an increase in undesirable practices such as cigarette and marijuana smoking.

In addressing the issues of social competence, then, family therapy truly becomes an ecological therapy: it can intervene in a variety of social systems that influence adolescent behavior and that may be helping to create or maintain dysfunctional social patterns.

ADOLESCENT NARCISSISM

Narcissism in adolescence is characterized by the adolescent thinking of him or herself as the focus of family attention. For the troubled adolescent, such narcissism produces a sense of omnipotence and the feeling that one does not have to accommodate to social realities and, therefore, does not have to change.

Family therapy deals with dysfunctional narcissism by attempting to create for the adolescent the experience of developmental estrangement. This experience consists of those moments of existential realization that the adolescent is on his own and must come to terms with the fact that Mom and Dad will not always salve his wounds, come to his rescue, or bail him out of difficult life situations. In this process the job of the family therapist is to monitor and support change as it occurs. Estrangement is an important goal of family therapy in that it obliges the adolescent to change. The shedding of adolescent narcissism and the acceptance of necessary change is part of maturation, and this, of course, is what family therapy is all about—helping the child to grow up.

SEPARATION

Growing up inevitably involves separation, the process through which the adolescent leaves home to become autonomous. Separation is a central task for all adolescents but often can become extremely stressful for both the adolescent and the family. Functional separation requires leaving without alienation, and this is one of the key goals of family therapy. To encourage a functional breaking away, the therapist must help not only with the separating adolescent but also with those people from whom he is separating. All of these individuals must gradually let go and then reconnect. Family therapy works to make this aching but rewarding process a reality.

Plan of the Book

In this chapter I have laid out what I believe to be the important issues of adolescence. In the one following I develop a therapeutic approach to adolescent difficulties. In addition, I introduce and explain some of the therapeutic and assessment tools I believe especially useful, among them the four-dimensional model and the identification of the homeostatic maintainer and the process parameters for brief therapy.

The developmental issues discussed in the opening chapters manifest themselves in behavioral problems for the troubled adolescent. The clinical chapters that follow illustrate approaches for dealing with and resolving such problems. Each clinical chapter covers a serious problem of adolescence: delinquency, runaway, violence, incest, suicide, and disability. These chapters include a discussion of the problem, principles of treatment, and a clinical case. Each case study includes the following: an assessment of the family and the goals of therapy; transcripts of one or more clinical sessions, annotated to highlight adolescent issues and therapeutic approaches; a case follow-up.* A summary of changes in the family that led to an amelioration of the problem is also given.

The final portion of the book deals with the parents as a subsystem and covers both single-parent and couple situations illustrated by appropriate clinical case studies. The final chapter reveals the results of a two-and-a-half-year follow-up of one of these families.

---

* The focus of this book is on what I identified as the turning points in therapy. Space limitations have precluded, in most cases, the inclusion of the work behind these turning points, i.e. the work with subsystems, the "chinese boxes" described in the next chapter. One important "box," or subsystem, is the therapist and the adolescent—together with siblings and maybe even peers. I believe it is important to do such work parallel to the family work. The therapist can function as a key transitional element in some of these systems until others—ideally immediate family members and peers—are seen as supportive enough to assume this function.

This subsystem therapy deals with individual issues—ones that the adolescent may not yet feel comfortable discussing with his or her parents, such as goals, motivation, and fears. *The family issues are not discussed.* If they were, then the sessions, much like safety valves, would diffuse pressure that instead is essential to drive the family to change: the therapist could undermine his or her own work with the family.

A question that always surfaces here: how to carry on a parallel therapy with the youngster—one that entails a contract for privileged information—and also work with the parents and the youngster in a context in which the youngster may be exposed? In my experience, participants have, with the exception of certain rare cases, understood that the therapist's allegiance is to a higher value, to the relationships and welfare of *all* participants. Families seem to understand the meta-rule that the therapist will move as is necessary for the safety of all.

2

The Tools of Therapy

Three umpires were having an argument about which of them was the best umpire. The first said, "I am the best because I calls 'em as I sees 'em." The second retorted, "I'm the best because I calls 'em the way they are." The third umpire, stepping back slightly from the other two, cried, "I'm the best umpire—because the balls, they ain't nothin' 'till I calls 'em."

—ALAN MACKAY

THE BEST THERAPIST, like the third umpire in the anecdote, acts to distinguish problems and thus to help create a more functional reality for the family. Just as the balls "ain't nothin' " until they are called, so the clinician must distinguish the specific therapeutic problem out of an almost limitless number of possibilities. Moreover, it is the responsibility of the therapist to persuade the family to accept the different and hopefully more functional reality that leads to a quick amelioration of problems. When working with adolescents, brief therapy is preferred because adolescents, like saplings, are experiencing rapid growth. If a sapling's angle of growth is corrected in time, the tree will grow straighter and stronger. So it is with adolescents. It is essential, therefore, for the therapist to assess the family situation correctly and to move to create a 'therapeutic reality' that will lead to the fastest transformation of the system. The tools introduced in the following pages are designed to help the therapist transform the family system as rapidly as possible and enable the family to stabilize a new, more functional structure.

Assessment Tools

The family therapist uses assessment tools to understand the nature of the family's organization and process as well as its strengths and weaknesses. In addition, these tools should help the therapist specify therapeutic goals and strategies.

THE FOUR-DIMENSIONAL MODEL

The detailed assessment approach that I use I call the four-dimensional model. This tool can help the therapist assess a family system from a number of different perspectives. The model is four-dimensional in several ways. First, there are four aspects of assessment for the therapist to consider: contemporary developmental pressures on the family, history, structure, and process. Furthermore, the process dimension is, as will be discussed later, an extra, or fourth, dimension that involves the subjective reaction of the therapist similar to the inclusion of a space-time perspective in physics or in painting.

The concept of four-dimensional space has, of course, been around for a long time. It revolutionized contemporary physics and has had profound effects in non-Euclidian mathematics and other fields such as painting. In cubist art, for example in Marcel Duchamp's famous *Nude Descending a Staircase*, the three dimensions of physical space are transformed by the fourth dimension of time, allowing the artist to portray the figure in motion from numerous angles. In my model, the transforming dimension is the therapist him- or herself. While the other therapeutic perspectives are linear and objective—the result of what the therapist observes in the treatment room—the fourth dimension is more subjective. It is determined both by the therapist's feelings when in the presence of the family and by the therapist's active participation in the very process of treatment.

The four-dimensional model should give the therapist, like the cubist painter, a kaleidoscopic view of his or her subject. It allows the therapist to look at a moving system from different perspectives. It also takes into consideration the therapist's position in the process as the therapist moves in and out of the system, sometimes as a neutral observer, other times as an involved protagonist who supports a particular family member or suddenly realizes the family's control. This emphasis on process and the therapist's active place in it is what helps define family therapy as a therapy of experience—with the therapy focusing first on the family's enactment of its dysfunctional patterns and then, later, on more functional, corrective ways of interacting. The four-dimensional model can help the therapist guide the family through this transformation.

Let us take a closer look now at the individual dimensions of the model. The first dimension is the *contemporary* developmental pressures that are destabilizing the family. Like all living systems, families have tendencies toward both equilibrium and evolution. During the course of a family's life, there are destabilizing developmental pressures that disrupt equilibrium and challenge the family to evolve. The therapist must be able to detect these points of instability, for these are times when the family's structural rules do not hold and, as Ilya Prigogine (in Minuchin and Fishman 1971, 21) says, the fluctuations created by developmental pressures can result in a dissipative state that is formed and maintained by non-equilibrium conditions leading to a new structure.

Destabilizing events create stress to which family systems can react in different ways. Some systems respond by transforming the rules under which they operate, thereby allowing new, more functional behaviors. In other systems, rather than changing shape, a medical or psychological symptom emerges.

The work of Holmes and Rahe (1967), confirming the association between stressful life events and illness leading to hospitalization, supports the clinical observation that patients who present medical and presumably psychological problems are living in a system in which some destabilizing factor has increased the stress on the family. The destabilizing factor may be positive or negative—a new baby, for example, or the death of a parent. It may be predictable or unpredictable—an older child leaving home or a child killed in an accident. Whatever the nature of the precipitating factor, at the emergence of the symptom these families become stuck and organize around the symptom so that the family members cannot address their developmental needs.

A powerful example of a symptomatic status quo caused by contemporary premises is discussed in chapter 5. In the violent family that is described, there were developmental pressures among both generations. The parents, who were in their early thirties, had the pressure of raising four children, three of whom were adolescents, as well their own issues of trying to attain educational and job skills they had missed as young parents. The teenagers, for their part, were struggling to develop their own competence and to function on their own. These pressures coalesced to produce behavior problems—drinking, violence, and poor performance in school and work—which became the focus of the family disruption. The result was a dysfunctional but stable situation in which the causative stress was not effectively dealt with.

The importance of this first dimension is that it informs the therapist of the developmental tasks with which the family is struggling. With this knowledge the therapist can design and direct the treatment necessary to help the family achieve its developmental goals.

The second dimension in the model involves the history of the system, the individual and family background that may contribute essential information regarding options to the therapy. The therapist must take the history of important events such as the death of a parent, the loss of a child, divorce, illness, a financial reversal, and so forth. The therapist must try to understand the history of the problem presented, the steps the family has taken to attempt its resolution, and the involvement of any other therapists, past and present. In addition, the therapist must try to ascertain biological processes such as organic brain syndrome or any other medical conditions.

The historical dimension is essential to the therapy because it provides information regarding the chronicity and severity of the family system's dysfunction. The family described in the clinical chapter on couples therapy (chapter 10) illustrates how significant the historical dimension can be. In this couple, the wife had been anorexic for more than twenty years. She abused laxatives, often taking a box at a time, and had been rushed to the hospital in a coma on several occasions. With historical data such as this, the therapist knows the necessity of working even more intensively than usual, as well as the importance of consulting closely with medical colleagues. A history is also important because it allows the therapist to garner vital information about the current concerns of the family. We should keep in mind, however, that the history that a family reports reflects only a partial reality, a selective chronicle edited by present concerns. Families scan their collective reflections, remembering and retelling what they are concerned about at the present.

The third assessment dimension is structure. Structural considerations for the therapist concern the organization and demarcation of the therapeutic system, including important relationships outside as well as within the family. The therapist must decide what, in effect, constitutes "the family"—the structure of important relationships that should be included in the treatment. The therapist must consider the relationship of the defined family system not only with extended family members but also with external systems affecting individual family members—school, social agencies, friends, and other therapists.

Later in this book we shall see how structure was a key dimension in the chapter on treating an incestuous family (chapter 6). In this case, a number of social systems were involved: the mother's therapist, the father's therapist, the children's therapists, and the court. On inquiry, all of these helpers differed on what should be done. The only point each of them agreed on, it seemed, was that the other agencies knew less. (I felt myself falling into the same divisive morass when I entered the therapy room to consult.)

The other important structural consideration for the therapist involves the issue of proximity and distance between the important figures in the system. The therapist assesses a family system on the basis of the appropriateness of the proximity and distance between members of the system at a given point in time of the family's development. The appropriateness is determined by considering the family life cycle and the resulting changes that have taken place in the family structure.

It is, of course, axiomatic in psychology that the family structure changes with the passage of time and that these changes tend to follow regular patterns. What is less widely recognized is that these changes are the result of the concurrent development of the children and the adults within the family system (Carter and McGoldrick 1980). As therapists we are aware of individual life cycles and look for the classic transitional stages of adolescence, courtship, marriage, having children, children leaving home, old age, and so forth. But we must also factor in those specific points of adult developmental crisis that are likely to occur within this classic life cycle—breaking away from parents, the age-forty crisis (which tends to occur in the thirties for blue-collar families), middle-age, and retirement. As pointed out by Gail Sheehy (1976) and Daniel J. Levinson and associates (1978), these adult crises tend to occur with the same regularity as do the developmental stages in children. The overlapping of individual child development, individual adult development with its attendant crises, and the development of the family as a unit can result in a shifting structural context. And in evaluating a family, the therapist must be aware of this shifting structure and be able to make the correct distinctions regarding appropriate proximity and distance. For example, a mother and son are only appropriately or inappropriately close in accordance with the developmental stages of child, adult, and family. A mother and three-day-old son who are inseparable are appropriately close. But if a mother and her seventeen-year-old son are inseparable, there is very likely a problem of inappropriate proximity.

Structure, then, is a key dimension in any therapeutic assessment of a family system. Its exploration can reveal to the therapist not only what the operant therapeutic unit is but also what is appropriate interaction within the unit according to the stages of development reached by individuals and by the family as a whole.

The fourth dimension is process. In assessment it is useful to keep in mind that descriptions of a system by family therapists are different from those done by anthropologists or novelists. Unlike our colleagues in these other fields, family clinicians do not maintain a fixed distance from the family. At times we may in fact become part of the system through techniques such as unbalancing, where the therapist acts as a protagonist in the family drama. During the session the therapist must be able to distance him- or herself from the events and describe the subjective experience of the system.

The process dimension involves the search for interactional patterns in the system. There are two types of patterns that must be assessed: patterns the therapist sees operating within the system and the therapist's own patterns of response. The first of these refers to transactional patterns, such as enmeshment or conflict diffusion, which the therapist can observe taking place in the treatment room. The second involves the more difficult area of the therapist's own subjective responses as one both intervenes within and withdraws from the system.

In the process of interaction with and disengagement from the family, the therapist will both act and be acted upon. In assessing the system, the therapist must be aware of interactional patterns of which he or she becomes a part. In addition, the therapist must recognize that to some extent one's reactions will be affected by one's own professional and personal contexts. For example, does the therapist have two supervisors who fervently espouse conflicting models? The therapist's assessments may also be affected by the therapist's own family context—family of origin, contemporary family system, spouse, children, and extended family.

Therapists bring into the treatment room, then, a number of subjective factors that can affect the assessment of family systems. By recognizing, and if necessary resisting, the pressures of their own contexts, by keeping in mind this "fourth dimension," therapists are both enlightened about the system and better prepared to evaluate the information they receive from and about families.

IDENTIFICATION OF THE HOMEOSTATIC MAINTAINER

I believe that one of the most useful assessment tools available to the family therapist is the concept of the homeostatic maintainer, the individuals or social forces that are maintaining a given problem and must therefore be included in the treatment.

The term *homeostatic maintainer* derives from the word *homeostasis* or *same state*. As used in biology or physiology, homeostasis refers to a process of maintaining sameness by restoring a system to a state from which it periodically departs. A classic example of a homeostatic mechanism is the thermotactic system in the human body. This system acts like a regulator to maintain body heat at a constant temperature to maximize efficiency both in cell reproduction and in interaction with the environment. As we know, however, there are times of crisis, such as infection or injury, when the critical function of the thermotactic system is to *raise* body temperature. During these periods, increased temperatures act to enhance the production of white blood cells and to destroy infecting agents. While the overall goal of the higher temperature is to improve bodily protection, if this excess heat is maintained for too long a period—if it becomes a new status quo—there can be deleterious side effects. The homeostatic system, then, can prove either a positive or a negative force.

With a family in crisis, there can be forces at work that act to maintain the status quo in a way that is detrimental to the system, by keeping the system from changing in the face of developmental pressures. It is this negative characteristic of homeostasis that makes it an important concept for family therapy. Like the body, the family system can include forces that keep it in a steady state that proves harmful because it prevents the family from adapting to developmental changes. The system either cannot allow a necessary increase in social "temperature" to deal with crisis, or it persists in crisis and cannot return to "normal"—to an everyday productive functioning.

A few years ago, the newspapers reported a story of a nineteen-year-old man who had committed an armed robbery in a rural community. When his court-appointed attorney went to see him, the man pulled a knife and held the young woman prisoner for three days. Finally the man was apprehended and had his day in court. When, just before sentencing, the judge asked, "Is there anything you would like to say in your own behalf?" the man remained silent but gestured to his mother. The middle-aged mother then stood, pointed to the judge, and said, "How dare you treat my son like this! It's not fair. He's done nothing wrong."

With just this brief story to go on, one can only guess about the true nature of the forces in the young man's life that had buffered him from facing the consequences of his actions. But it is clear that even at this eleventh hour, in the face of overwhelming evidence of culpability, the mother refused to hold her son responsible and instead acted to maintain the status quo. This was a family system held fast in negative homeostasis, where productive change had not been allowed and where terrible dysfunction had come to be accepted as the norm.

The family therapist uses the concept of the homeostatic maintainer by attempting to render ineffective the family's stereotyped, stable ways of responding. The first step for the therapist is to discover what is maintaining the problem—that is, the person or persons who are encouraging the homeostasis—then distinguish a therapeutic unit that includes the homeostatic maintainer. The therapist must obviously demarcate the extent of the forces to be worked with—mother, father, grandparents, neighbors, teachers. As Francisco Varela (1976) points out, family systems can be like Chinese boxes: individuals are part of a family, which is part of an extended family, which is part of a community, and so forth. The job of the therapist is to identify and focus on the "box" that may hold the homeostatic maintainer and then treat this unit as the family system. The second step in the treatment process is for the therapist to disrupt the system and observe who attempts to return the system to its status quo. That person or social force is the homeostatic maintainer.

A very clear example of a family member functioning as a homeostatic maintainer is the father described in the chapter on delinquency (chapter 3). Early in the session, when his wife was confronting their delinquent youngster (who had been caught the night before with some of her jewelry and an empty vial of cocaine), the father, by his passivity and solicitous concern for his son, continually undermined his wife's efforts to have the boy respond to parental authority. He sat passively and stared at his son while his wife confronted the adolescent. By not joining with his wife in the confrontation, the father was implying approval and thus maintaining the dysfunctional pattern of the boy's illegal behavior.

IDENTIFICATION OF KEY TRANSACTIONAL PATTERNS

Once the therapist has assessed the individuals or forces maintaining the problem, the next step is to identify the patterns that are contributing to dysfunction in the system. The therapist's goal here is to make use of these patterns to map out a strategy for brief therapy, a treatment that will produce the fastest possible change. Other therapies—such as psychoanalysis, cognitive therapies, and behaviorism—provide a tremendous array of possible descriptions of individual and family problems. But our interest here is not to describe the family in all of its complexity. After all, therapy is neither anthropology nor literature; it is changing systems. And to do this with the greatest efficiency we must look for the most parsimonious description, the identification of the patterns that will allow for the most rapid change.

There are a number of key patterns that the therapist should look for. One is certainly conflict avoidance. Dysfunctional families often take steps to bypass confrontation and avoid acknowledging conflict. For example, a therapist may bring up a difficult issue and ask the parents to discuss it with each other, only to find that they are so persistent in avoiding confrontation between themselves that instead they direct their response entirely to the therapist or to their children, retreating to safe ground whenever possible.

For example, in the chapter on runaways (chapter 4) the parents in the case study allowed their 15-year-old daughter to leave home rather than enforcing their rules. At the time of the session the girl was living with an 18-year-old boy in a very tough neighborhood. In the therapy room the parents seemed like two magnetic poles, repelling each other as I challenged them to resolve their differences and take some action to retrieve their daughter from potential danger.

Other patterns that therapists may well encounter in dysfunctional families include complementary and symmetrical schizmogenesis. (Bateson 1972). The term *schizmogenesis* refers to escalating sequences of interaction leading to a schism. In its complementary form, this pattern can be observed as a series of reciprocal-fitting behaviors. For example, a therapist might encounter a wife who is angry and a husband who complains of stomachaches. When the pattern escalates, the wife becomes angrier and the husband has escalated to the point where he has a bleeding ulcer. In the symmetrical form, the individuals act in concert. For example, there may be a heated argument in which neither party can back down. When this pattern escalates, violence may erupt on both sides.

There are additional patterns that may be observed in certain families, such as psychosomatic families (Minuchin, Rosman, and Baker 1978). Here the therapist is likely to encounter patterns like enmeshment. This is an extreme form of proximity and intensity in family interactions, resulting in both poorly differentiated boundaries between family members and a lack of proper distinctions in the perceptions those family members have of one another and of themselves. I remember seeing Salvador Minuchin at work with a psychosomatic family in which the lack of boundaries of the enmeshed family was very evident. In the therapy room are father, mother, and 12-year-old diabetic daughter. Minuchin walks into the room and squeezes the girl's arm, asking the father, "Can you feel that?" The father replies, "You know, it's odd, I can feel that!" Minuchin then asks the mother the same question. Mother: "I can't feel that, but I have poor circulation."

Another pattern often encountered in psychosomatic families is rigidity. This refers to the inability of families to depart from the status quo when circumstances would seem to necessitate change. Such families remain committed to accustomed patterns of interaction and resist change. This is especially problematic for families with adolescents, where issues of the adolescent's autonomy are apt to stress the usual rules of family interaction. The chapter in this book on the suicidal adolescent (chapter 7) deals in depth with this type of rigid family. The suicidal child is living in a family where there is such severe rigidity that the only way to be heard, to communicate that things need to change, is to commit the ultimate act of desperation. Frequently these families are ones that make fixed demands on the child; their message is: "You are valued for what you *do*, not for *being you*." Another frequently seen pattern is a rigid stance that communicates a message to the adolescent that says, "No matter how hard you try, the family does not want you."

Overprotectiveness is yet another pattern that may be found in psychosomatic and other families. The degree of concern family members have for one another is exaggerated, often preventing a child from developing autonomy and competence. An interesting case of overprotectiveness is discussed in the chapter on disability (chapter 8). In this family a 19-year-old, mildly retarded Swedish girl was living in a system that was organized to provide for her every need. This system was possible because the family lived in a social environment where there was a great abundance of services to assist them. The family and the outside helpers would not allow the young woman to try to become more independent. When seen after her cautious suicide attempt, the girl confided that she desperately wanted to try to get a job, live away from home, and manage her own money. These might have been simple and attainable needs, but the overprotective system would not let her attempt to stretch her abilities and grow to achieve her goals.

Many families that exhibit patterns of enmeshment, rigidity, and overprotectiveness also demonstrate an inability to cope directly with conflict. As a result, a pattern of conflict diffusion is common in such families. Conflict is diffused through the activation and complementary focusing of a family member, often the symptomatic adolescent. The result is an inability to confront differences and negotiate satisfactory resolutions.

Conflict avoidance and conflict diffusion differ only in that the latter is a term used to describe what can actually happen during a family therapy session. When tension begins to build between two people, a third person attempts to reduce the tension. For example, in the case study in chapter 5, when the father and the eldest son began to argue during the session, the next eldest son chimed in and complained that he wanted to be heard. What made it clear that this was a pattern of conflict diffusion and not just the boy's spontaneous need to be heard was the fact that at virtually every time conflict seemed about to emerge, one or another family member would interrupt, and the net effect was that the conflict would be forgotten.

These patterns of psychosomatic family organization are frequently seen, in part or entirely, in families that present problems other than psychosomatic ones. Patterns such as these, as well as the others mentioned, must be addressed for the therapy to be brief. These are pivotal patterns that can be observed and changed in the therapy room. And as long as therapy is directed toward these fundamental patterns, the treatment can move forward rapidly. Conversely, if these patterns are not being altered in the therapy, the clinician should conclude that it is time to change strategies.

Essential Techniques

The family therapy orientation of this book is based on the specific techniques described in much greater depth in *Family Therapy Techniques*, by Minuchin and Fishman (1981). There are many therapeutic techniques in structural family therapy that are useful in working with adolescents and their families. Those discussed in the following paragraphs, however, are some of the therapeutic tools that I have found most helpful in transforming dysfunctional adolescent family systems.

BOUNDARY MAKING

Boundary making is the cornerstone of family therapy with adolescents. The central issue of achieving a separate identity in preparation for leaving home depends on how well a family deals with boundaries. When the therapist works with boundary making, to either attenuate or bolster existing boundaries around subsystems, he/she is working with the pivotal interactional process. A definition of boundary making includes the process by which the therapist helps to control membership of family members in subsystems. The therapist may encourage participation of subsystem members with other family members as well as with the extra-familial system or the therapist may also exclude members. The therapist may do this by increasing proximity and experimentation among the sub-system members.

Of course, interpersonal boundaries do not exist, visually speaking. They are a construction to help the therapist describe patterned transactions among family members with the exclusion of other family members. Boundaries define both the members that are included as well as those that are excluded. And they are described from a continuum of enmeshed to disengaged. How functional a given boundary is depends on the developmental stage of a youngster, as mentioned earlier.

ENACTMENT

Enactment involves the therapist's encouraging interpersonal scenarios during the treatment session in which the dysfunctional transactions among family members are played out. The effective use of enactment usually consists of three steps. In step one the therapist observes the spontaneous transactions of the family and decides which dysfunctional areas to highlight. In the second step the therapist organizes the scenarios and allows the dysfunctional process to be played out, perturbing the system when necessary to increase intensity. In the third step the therapist challenges ways of transacting till more functional transactional patterns emerge, and the process of therapeutic change begins. *For enactment to occur the therapist must assume a decentralized position.*

This technique of enactment distinguishes family therapy from other therapies. Its focus is on the provocation, assessment, and amelioration of interactional patterns between significant people in the adolescent's life that can be observed in the actual process of therapy. Such techniques are normally not used in psychoanalysis, cognitive therapy, or behaviorism. And while in gestalt therapy the clinician may indeed focus on patterns, the patterns emerge between relative strangers, not between actual family members who go home and live their lives in some proximity.

The enactment technique is a powerful tool for family therapists. It allows the therapist to see the problem in operation as well as to see change. This is especially useful in cases such as those involving patterns of violence. The logicians tell us that one cannot prove a negative. One cannot prove that violence will not recur. But if one follows the progression of new family patterns in therapy and sees new, more functional transactions taking place in the treatment room, then one can be reasonably sure that the old patterns will not recur. It is this insistence on "show me," that makes the technique so effective. A fundamental principle of this therapy is that if the therapist cannot see changes, there is no way of assuring that they have in fact occurred. Reports of people "feeling better" are evanescent; enactment of change and seeing new family interactional patterns stabilize make a far better gauge of successful therapy.

UNBALANCING

Unbalancing is a technique in which the therapist challenges and changes the family organization. When using this technique the therapist, rather than presenting a balanced, "firm but fair" point of view, joins the family system and acts to support only one individual or subsystem. For example, the therapist may affiliate with a family member low in hierarchy and help empower that person; or the therapist may form coalitions with certain family members to confront another member of the system. The object is to change the usual signals that direct the interpersonal behavior within the family. With new signals provoked by the therapist's affiliation, family members may act in unaccustomed ways and may feel free to explore unfamiliar possibilities for personal and interpersonal functioning.

The unbalancing technique can be quite effective in altering power alliances within a system. However, unbalancing makes unique, at times uncomfortable, demands on the therapist. For one thing, it calls upon the therapist to break with tradition and take sides. With unbalancing, the therapist uses an accrued position within the system in an unexpected way that may produce stress for both family and therapist alike. In addition, the therapist must be careful not to be inducted into the family's dysfunctional pattern, suddenly becoming a kind of henchman who reinforces instead of disrupts old behaviors. This technique can be especially difficult when working with adolescents because the therapist may frequently have to "work both sides of the street," alternately supporting child and parents in a shifting pattern of coalitions.

REFRAMING

The technique of reframing involves the therapeutic introduction of alternative realities that provide family members with a different framework for experiencing themselves and one another. The therapist offers a different reality and the therapy then evolves from a clash of old and new realities. The family's framing is designed for the continuity and maintenance of its current system. The therapeutic framing is intended to move the family toward a reworking of the dysfunctional reality. Out of this clash of realities, then, the therapist looks not only for changed cognition but also for the *emergence of different interactional patterns*. The emphasis is on changed interaction leading to new understanding as well as to changed experience, both in the treatment room and at home.

SEARCH FOR COMPETENCE

Another key technique for the therapist is the search for competence in all family members, the object being to expand alternatives and help individuals discover new, more positive selves. As mentioned in the preceding chapter, one of the underlying rules of family therapy is its insistence on the multifaceted self—on the great potential for functional possibilities within dysfunctional individuals and systems. The goal in the search for competence, then, is both to confirm the individual and to challenge the system that is preventing the emergence of more positive, more functional behavior.

INTENSITY

In order to produce change in a family system the therapist must, of course, first be able to get his or her message across. In even the most highly motivated of troubled families the therapist's message may never register. There is, in a sense, a family threshold of deafness that must be overcome. In order to make a family "hear," the therapist uses intensity, the technique of selectively regulating the degree of feeling in the room in order to amplify the therapeutic message. The variations in intensity can be wide, from simple, low-key communications to high-intensity crises. The appropriate level will depend on the family's readiness for response and on the level of the homeostatic threshold. Below this threshold the family may simply deflect or assimilate information without really getting the message. As therapists we should always remember that information sent is not necessarily information received. The therapist can be sure that the family has received only when different patterns begin to emerge in the room. It is the therapist's job to constantly monitor the intensity, increasing the level until the family's threshold is surpassed and new behavior becomes evident.

These are some of the tools, both assessment and therapeutic, that I have found most useful in addressing the problems of families with troubled adolescents. In the clinical chapters that follow I show how these tools can be used to evaluate dysfunction and stimulate change in actual families in treatment.

PART II

TREATING DISTURBANCES OF ADOLESCENTS: CLINICAL CASES

3

Treating Delinquency: Addressing the Premises of Self

In wolves and dogs there is a close association between mothers and puppies during the first three weeks of life. After this period, and at the time when the mother leaves the litter for long periods, the strongest relationships are formed with litter mates. This is the basis of pack organization of adult dogs and wolves.

—JOHN PAUL SCOTT

SALVADOR MINUCHIN (1967) notes that Eskimos will steal newborn wolf puppies away from their mothers before they have reached three weeks of age in order to develop an "unwolf-like wolf," nurturing it as they would nurture a human child. Minuchin uses this example to illustrate an essential truth in the treatment of adolescent delinquents: that the origins of the problem do not reside solely in a triangular dysfunction between parental figures and the delinquent. In addition to troubled relationships between parents and child and the developmental stresses within the adolescent, the therapist must also address the effects of an external system of peers, siblings, and others who can dramatically influence the adolescent. This chapter deals with the treatment of delinquent adolescents, the family systems involved, and the external system of both peers and adults—extended family members, siblings, friends, court officers, and others—that may contribute to maintaining delinquent behavior.

The Growing Problem of Delinquency

Delinquency, defined as crimes reported to police that are committed by juveniles, has increased considerably since World War II. Since the late 1960s the rate of juvenile delinquency has risen even more sharply, with a particularly marked rise in violent crime and crimes associated with drug use and prostitution. This rise in crime is not gender specific. In fact, the increase in crime rate for fourteen to seventeen-year-old girls since 1957 has been even greater than that for boys. In 1957 the ratio of male to female crimes was 10.79 to 1; by 1977 it had fallen to 4.97 to 1 (Rutter 1980). It is apparent that criminal delinquency is one field where equal opportunity has become a reality. One might, of course, ponder the accuracy of these and other statistics related to juvenile crime, since the determination and reporting of delinquency may in some cases be affected by the political climate of the communities involved. Nevertheless, it is clear that juvenile delinquent behavior is an increasingly serious problem.

During the last thirty years there have been great changes in family life. The traditional three-generational, vertical family has been gradually replaced by the horizontal organization of parent(s), friends, and helpers. And even this horizontal system has been undergoing more flux than the vertical system did in previous generations.

One result of the family's becoming a more unstable institution is that the adolescent both turns to and is more influenced by peers and siblings. Salvador Minuchin and associates (1967), in their seminal study of one hundred delinquent boys at the Wiltwyck School for Boys in New York City, found that, in the families of delinquents, siblings were very significant in the development of self-concept. This does not necessarily mean that parental figures are completely eclipsed; they remain extremely important. But these researchers found that to the extent that the parental subsystem is weak, there is an effective relinquishing of parental authority, and the result is that the sibling subsystem becomes even more powerful.

If there is any one characteristic common to families with delinquents, it is that parental authority has been weakened in some way. In their work at Wiltwyck, Minuchin and his colleagues found many families in which either there was no actual father figure or, if he was present, the male was most often a transient figure. In this second category, the father tended to delegate the rearing and education of the children completely to the mother, as if these areas of development were the mother's exclusive province. In families in which a single woman was raising the children, often the mother was able to respond and interact with her children only when they were submissive or requesting that some basic need be met. In these families the maternal motto seemed to be "I am available." But in reality this availability did not include effective executive guidance.

There are many other patterns of weakened parental authority. In some families the parental figures are ineffective not because they are uncomfortable in exerting parental guidance but because there is a chronic pattern of disagreement between the parents that renders them ineffective. The disagreement, or split, can exist between any combination of parental figures. The parents may be present in the home but in chronic disagreement with one parent overinvolved with one of the children, often the delinquent. Or the disabling split may be between a parent and grandparent, or between the social agency and the court that are responsible for the adolescent. Whatever the split or splits, the result is the same ineffective executive authority that leaves adolescents to search for guidance on their own, wherever they can find it.

What is the best way to address this problem of delinquency? The biological event of adolescence has not changed perceptibly over the last forty years. Since nature has not changed, nurture must have. Social changes are therefore seen to be responsible for this phenomenon. Thus, an appropriate therapy must address both the delinquent child and the social matrix that is maintaining the problem behavior.

I propose that contextual therapy is the most effective treatment. There have been a number of studies that support this view. For example, work done by Scott W. Henggeler and associates (1986) reveals that delinquent adolescents who received family therapy evidenced significant decreases in conduct problems, anxious-withdrawn behaviors, immaturity, and association with delinquent peers. In addition, the mother-adolescent and marital relations in the families of these adolescents became significantly warmer, and the adolescent became much more involved in family interaction. In contrast, families with delinquents who received alternative treatment evidenced no positive changes and showed deterioration in affective relations.

The significance of such studies is their demonstration that when the family is treated as a unit, increased warmth and affection result, which in turn lead to a changed role for the adolescent in the family. Prior to treatment the adolescents were at best disengaged from the family and at worst in open conflict with one or both parents. After treatment there was increased positive reciprocity among all family members. Clearly, then, this kind of therapy represents the most promising means of reconstituting a functional family system as well as providing for the adolescent's nondelinquent development. All too often the troubled adolescent's context does not challenge either the behavior or the premises of self that support delinquency. An effective therapy must confront both.

General Principles

EXAMINING THE PREMISES OF SELF

In my discussion of the homeostatic maintainer in chapter 2, I relate the story of a mother defending her delinquent son in the face of overwhelming evidence of guilt. This was a classic case of a parent contributing to delinquency by acting to maintain a dysfunctional status quo. Uncovering and transforming homeostatic mechanisms is only a first step in work with delinquents. The process must go further and address the deterioration that has taken place in the adolescent's emerging self. As Gregory Bateson notes, "the essence of the delinquency is not the breaking of rules, but . . . the fact that . . . premises for conducting [oneself] as a rule breaker are not touched by the outside" (quoted in Hampden-Turner 1982, 145). In other words, the delinquent is living in a system organized in such a way that "the outside" does not affect the delinquent's premises. The delinquent merely says to himself, "It was a failure. Next time I won't get caught." The premises underlying the behavior have not been touched.

TRANSFORMING THE PREMISES BEHIND THE BEHAVIOR

Clearly, without a therapy that changes the premises of the self, we cannot change the delinquent. We may suppress the personality, but we will not affect the delinquency. In order to transform rather than merely interrupt the delinquency, we need a therapy that will help structure more functional premises for behavior.

I think we seldom fully achieve it. Most of the time what we do is to retard, suppress, or lessen the frequency of delinquent behavior. This is not a dishonorable role, but neither is it enough. It is important to continue the therapy so that the adolescent can become attached to a more functional context that will call forth areas of competence, which in turn will confirm the nondelinquent self.

We must constantly think in terms of how the therapy can foster these more functional contexts. We must assume that even in situations of chronic delinquency, where moral development has been severely impaired, there exists a nascent, better self that can be reached within a context that allows an expression of competence. We must posit that before becoming delinquent the adolescent must have had some experience with this good self, the self that could make choices and exercise competence. Tapping into this, however, is often a struggle because it may be that the delinquent peer community is the only place where the adolescent is perceived as competent. In that context, then, the delinquent self is the self that can "do." The struggle is to transfer this competence to other, nondelinquent areas.

Most of the time, however, the competent self simply is not available in any existing context. The youngster has had to go totally underground and has developed an anti-establishment self. Often, to discover what nurtures and enlivens the self, the therapist must search the garden where the delinquent has been watered: the world of the delinquent's peers. Working with this external, second family may be more effective than treating the family that shares room and board with the adolescent. This counter-context may reveal the vitality and excitement that the delinquent receives from the delinquency and that prolongs it in the absence of competence.

PREVENTING THE PARENTS FROM BEING DEFEATED

Maintaining the balance of forces is essential to family therapy, and one concept is key to its maintenance: the parents must not be defeated. They must continue to exercise their function of executive controller. But this alone is never sufficient. The parents must also emerge as executive nurturer, offering support and allowing the youngster to negotiate and to feel competent. Of course, if the child's main context is already fixed outside the family, the parents' rule can be undermined and their leverage eroded. In such cases the therapist's challenge is twofold: to attempt to recreate an intact parental hierarchy to balance the pull from peers and, at the same time, to try to use the external context—the world of peers—to strengthen the "good self" of the adolescent and reintroduce this competent self into the family. This double challenge is a difficult one for the therapist. The focus must be on creating experiences both within and outside the family to help mobilize positive behaviors and premises. In creating such experiences, the therapist will begin by generating intensity in the family system in order to bring dysfunctional patterns to the surface. The therapist might also choose to work with both family and peers to challenge conceptions of responsibility and honesty, in an attempt to build an ethical awareness in place of a concern for immediate material advantage alone. Often it is necessary for the therapist to make use of the developmental estrangement technique, to shock the delinquent out of the comfortable illusion that someone, usually Mom and Dad, will always be there to bail the youngster out of difficult situations.

ACTING QUICKLY TO INTERRUPT THE DELINQUENCY

Whatever techniques one chooses to employ, it is essential that the therapist act quickly to interrupt and challenge the delinquency. It is common for delinquent patterns to become entrenched over time. Therefore, it is critical that a therapeutic crisis be created as soon as possible in the course of therapy. Furthermore, care must be taken at the outset to include all essential members of the delinquent system, both from inside and outside the family. The therapist must then address this larger context and attempt to create a more therapeutic system, one that helps the internal monitors—the parents—evaluate and, to some extent, shape the influential external force of the peers.

CONFIRMING AREAS OF COMPETENCE

The key to defeating delinquency is to help the adolescent locate a context where a good, more competent self can emerge, so that when the youngster experiments with delinquency he is not pulled in totally and understands "being good" as an alternative. Then at least the premise of good behavior will have been established. If the family does not have enough benevolence or enough care and concern for the child, then strengthening the family's control will obviously serve only to contain the problem behavior. Eventually the youngster will slip back into delinquency. The therapy can attempt to transform the family context in many ways, but unless the premise for a good self has been created, nothing will really be accomplished.

It is encumbent upon the therapist when working with the parents and adolescent to find specific productive situations that maintain the "good self." This new environment will support the adolescent as competent. Thus he will receive confirmation from a different, nondelinquent set of peers.

Clinical Example: Carl, an Inveterate Delinquent

The case that follows illustrates what I think are critical processes in the shaping of the delinquent personality. The focus is on the interactional characteristics of the family, particularly the conflict between the adults, their inability to close ranks, and the reciprocal mistrust that prevents them from understanding or controlling the troublesome adolescent.

The family discussed here was presented to me by a therapist, one of my trainees, because he felt the system was not changing. The family members would agree and agree, but nothing would change. The therapist felt the family was engaged in a downward spiral and heading toward disaster. Carl, the sixteen-year-old son, was precocious in only one way: he was well beyond his years in criminality and delinquency. By age sixteen he had not only been selling cocaine for two years: he was also involved with considerably older professional drug dealers. Moreover, the young man was in debt to the drug dealers and the family was very much afraid that retribution would be taken against their home or other family members.

As we saw earlier in this chapter, the first step is to transform the system so that the immediate maintainers of the delinquency are curtailed. The therapist must then work to create a new context in which more functional areas of the adolescent's self will be supported. As in all of the cases presented in this book, in order to ascertain who or what was the homeostatic maintainer, I started with a full assessment of the system.

ASSESSMENT USING THE FOUR-DIMENSIONAL MODEL

History

Carl, a juvenile delinquent, was the last of five children from a suburban Philadelphia family. His older siblings ranged in age from twenty-five down; one sister was an accomplished graduate student in chemistry while one brother was unemployed and still living at home. Carl had been involved with drugs and stealing for close to two years. His father was a salesman for a pharmaceutical company, which led me to hypothesize that, in terms of symptom selection, conflict was diffused when the family focused on this specific behavior: selling drugs. It was interesting, but not surprising, that the young man's delinquency was a corollary of the father's occupation.

Carl was not living at home; at the suggestion of the therapist, he was staying with a friend. However, on the night before the session he was caught by his mother leaving his parents house with an empty vial of cocaine and some of her best silver.

Development

Carl was the last child, so the parental system had to reorganize around having no dependent children in the home. The mother and father were older parents, nearing retirement and faced with the prospect of having more time on their hands. They drove into their sessions from the New Jersey shore. The father was decreasing his work hours and focusing much more on his family. More immediately, with additional time at home he was faced with a smoldering conflict in his marriage that he had been trying to avoid for many years. That conflict was exacerbated by the fact that his wife was resentful of her husband's greater presence in the home, feeling that her space was being intruded upon.

Like all adolescents, Carl was insecure in terms of potential accomplishments and had one foot in and one out of the family life. He was untested and felt unsure about his ability to meet the growing demands that were being placed on him as he matured.

Structure

The family was profoundly split on how to deal with their delinquent son. The parents were in perpetual disagreement, and this disagreement was magnified by the presence of the father's father, with whom he was very close. The grandfather regularly gave his son advice, not only on what to do with Carl but also on how he should treat his wife. The parents' lack of agreement was confusing to their son. One parent might opt to be stern, while the other would decide to be more lenient. Then, much to Carl's (and perhaps the parents') amazement, their positions would flip-flop, the lenient parent choosing to be tough and the tough parent going into retreat. Of course, the effect of their inconsistency on Carl was to produce bewilderment and cynicism.

Process

This family was reminiscent of a psychosomatic system. There was extreme rigidity, enmeshment, conflict avoidance, and a diffusion of conflict via the activation of a third person. Throughout the session, at which I was present in the position of consultant, I found myself struggling to get the parents to talk together about any issue. When they would begin, one or the other would attempt to pull in the son, me, or the therapist. Alternately, either myself or the therapist or the son would spontaneously activate, diffusing tension.

My own experience in the room was one of frustration. I saw the overprotectiveness and conflict avoidance in the system as emasculating this boy's potential. At the same time I had to fight the urge to be either very polite or outrageous (the latter, I must confess, was the stronger urge). There was an almost palpable tension in the room.

The difficulty, then, was to get the parents to address each other in a different manner. To create immediate change I decided to intervene as I would in the family of an anorexic, using a classic approach to working with anorexics in which the family has lunch with the anorexic youngster in the therapy room. The therapist then tells the parents that it is their responsibility to get the child to eat so that the child will stay alive. This creates a therapeutic crisis which acts as a kind of fulcrum around which more functional patterns emerge. In this case the parents of the delinquent boy were instructed to search their child and, if necessary, call the police. In both cases the scenario challenges the conflict avoidance, the split between the parents, the triadic functioning, and the overprotectiveness. I believe these were the pivotal points—the joints in the family system.

The assessment led to some useful insights. First, this was a case in which normal adolescent ambivalence was greatly exaggerated by the family system. The inability of the parents to speak with one voice caused a split in Carl, the object of their disagreement. He was attached to and loved both parents, but if he heeded one he risked alienating the other. The parental split definitely reinforced the boy's ambivalence.

Carl's ambivalence was also underscored by his relations with siblings and peers. Two of his older siblings demonstrated opposing pulls. The successful graduate student was following in her father's footsteps and embarking on a career in sales; meanwhile, the unemployed brother who was drinking excessively was a negative presence in the home. The same split was evident in Carl's peers. Some of his peers remained in school and aspired to enter the mainstream culture; others, however, were part of a delinquent subculture. Carl found himself caught between these divergent influences of both siblings and peers, amplifying the normal stress associated with adolescent ambivalence.

Another valuable insight to be gained from our assessment was the extent to which this system encouraged symptomatic behavior in the adolescent as a way of maintaining homeostasis. It was evident that the parental conflict was being diffused by the focus on the delinquency symptoms of the child. This focus relieved stress on the parents but also kept them from addressing their own issues. This pattern was exaggerated by the parents' approaching retirement age. As the father became less involved with outside activities, the system needed the son to provide symptomatic behavior in order to stabilize the status quo. Had the parents been more involved with their respective pursuits, they would have had less energy and the system would probably have had less need for their son to be symptomatic. These assumptions are based on a theory of conservation of interest. Given that people have limited attention to expend in any particular direction, if family members have their interests happily employed elsewhere there will be less attention available to the symptomatic child. And the less attention paid to the symptoms, the less they will be reinforced. Of course, this is a vicious circle which emanates from and maintains the marital split.

THE THERAPY

The clinical goals of the therapy were as follows:

- To strengthen the parental dyad so that the parents would no longer be split and would communicate better with each other, resolve conflict between themselves, and function as effective executives in meting out negative (as well as positive) consequences for their son's delinquent behavior.
- To have conflict emerge and be resolved in the treatment room.
- To include other members of the system—siblings, peers, extended family— so that these members would not act to support the delinquency.
- To touch the pivotal structural dimensions of the adolescent and provoke an experience of developmental estrangement, addressing the fundamental premises of self.
- To encourage the family members to accept one another's positive selves so that a mutual liking could be established.
- To assist the adolescent in finding a supportive extrafamilial context that would reinforce his nondelinquent self, thus further addressing the fundamental premises of self.

Uncovering the Homeostatic Maintainer

The sequence that follows demonstrates my assessment of the homeostatic maintainer. I began by observing the family from behind a mirror.* The mother, blond and very thin, dressed fashionably in a pleated skirt and vest, was in her early fifties; the father, sixty and overweight, was wearing a plaid business suit. Carl was in black jeans and a black leather engineer's jacket and lizard skin boots. At this point I was searching for who or what was keeping this system developmentally stuck. The mother was in the process of explaining what had happened the night before, when she caught her son with an empty vial of cocaine and some of her silver.

MOTHER: He was going with a friend of his who I have some confidence in, so I thought, well, he's in pretty good hands—relatively sensible. I knew he was spending some length of time upstairs, so I said, "Before you leave the house, let me check your pockets." And I went through that jacket and I found a package—I assumed it was cocaine. I just assumed it was empty and I threw it on the counter. He has about one hundred zippers on his jacket, and I went through all those and I also found some silver of mine that apparently you (*speaking to Carl*) couldn't get any money for.

CARL: I gave it to you.

Carl qualifies his mother's statement with the premise that if he had given it to her, it is still his and he can take it away. In this case Carl expresses a conventional, classic phenomenology of the delinquent self.

MOTHER: After I got it out of your pocket you gave it to me. Well, that's beside the point. Whatever—you gave it to me, I found it—it was something that apparently you couldn't get any money for. . . .

CARL: You shouldn't be talking like this here (*pointing to the mirror*).

MOTHER: Carl, I don't think I'm hiding anything.

* In this, as in some of the other case studies dealt with in subsequent chapters, I was acting as consultant to a therapist in front of a supervisory group of about 8 to 10 trainees who observed the sessions from behind a one-way mirror; I would come in and out of the therapy session or call in to give the therapist suggestions.

At this point I entered the room because I felt that they were just reenacting previous sessions. I thought the system needed more intensity—more energy in a slightly different direction—as a response to the emergence of potentially powerful content: the theft from his mother as well as the empty vial of cocaine. What I had in mind was to act on the notion of homeostasis as a dynamic principle: that one must examine homeostasis at times of disequilibrium and observe how the system responds to perturbation. In this instance, I saw the cocaine and the stealing as potential perturbations and was curious to discover how the family responded.

What I was attempting to do was to uncover the key premises of this adolescent's self. The parental coddling was reinforcing Carl's idea that he was entitled to eternal forgiveness and that he could always con those to whom he was responsible. This family had no core concept of the parents as rule makers or enforcers. The direction of the therapy had to be to reorder some fundamental premises—not just to put the parents back in charge but also to change how the participants thought about themselves. The executives had to come to feel that they were not fools, and the young man had to realize that his parents had actual power. My concern was to arrange the transaction so that these ideas could surface and so that new selves for all participants could then emerge.

In this case Carl's latest misbehavior was old news to the family. As such, it did not represent a true destabilizing event. Yet the therapeutic team had to use it to stress the system as a means of revealing the compensatory responses that maintained the homeostasis. I therefore tried to create a crisis by focusing on the enormity of the boy's action and the inert reaction of the parents. By focusing, framing, and intensifying, the therapist can create a crisis that will disequilibrate the system. Once this happens the evident homeostatic processes can be examined and then worked with.

DR. FISHMAN: I am Dr. Fishman; I just want to ask you a question. I've spent about an hour talking about your history, your family. Not just about Carl, but about your whole family. I'll tell you something that absolutely amazes me. That is—I'm not even going to tell you what it is until you answer the question. When you found something that you presumed was cocaine and you also found silver that was stolen from you, what did the police say when you called them?

MOTHER: I did not call the police.

DR. FISHMAN: You see, that's the thing that we heard about your family and that's something that I find really extraordinary. (*To the father:*) What would happen to you if they found cocaine in your presence?

FATHER: If who found cocaine in my presence?

We see the first of the homeostatic mechanisms. By not calling the police, the family accommodated their son's misbehavior instead of ensuring negative consequences for his delinquency. To the extent that they accommodated, nothing changed. This response further solidified Carl's fundamental premise about himself: that he was invulnerable and could "handle" his parents.

DR. FISHMAN: If the police found that you had cocaine anywhere around you.

FATHER: I would probably lose my job and I certainly couldn't work for a drug company again.

DR. FISHMAN: How about if it were found in your home?

FATHER: I'd probably be in trouble.

DR. FISHMAN: You might even lose your livelihood?

FATHER: Very possibly.

DR. FISHMAN: Are you very wealthy and it doesn't matter?

FATHER: No, no—I'm just struggling.

DR. FISHMAN: Like all of us. So I don't understand why you didn't call the police.

The purpose of emphasizing the consequences for the family of being caught with cocaine was to increase the intensity by stressing the seriousness of what Carl was doing. I also wanted to challenge the family norm of accommodation to Carl, a pattern that was crippling to the boy. If the family was going to be helpful to their son they had to provide rules; they had to see to it that Carl was not bailed out but instead forced to be competent and law abiding. Furthermore, the rules of the family had to be made to replicate those of the outside world. The boy had to know that one faces consequences as a result of one's actions.

In the next sequence the homeostatic mechanisms emerge clearly. When the father agrees with me on the potential enormity of the difficulty, the mother interrupts to defuse the situation.

MOTHER: May I back up? I did not open the package. I assumed it was empty.

The mother's unwillingness to address the issue of her son's severe drug usage helps to maintain the problem. Of course she knew what was in the vial. Perhaps even more important, however, is the process. The father agrees that this episode is very serious, but the mother cuts him off and says she is not certain that it even happened. The father's focus on the seriousness of the offense distances him from Carl, while the mother gives Carl the benefit of the doubt and implicitly supports him. My job is to stress for the parents the potential consequences to themselves when they bail their son out. Part of the delinquent system is that the parents often behave as though they could escape the consequences of their children's delinquency.

DR. FISHMAN: Okay, but you knew what it was.

MOTHER: Well, I knew what the container was, but I didn't realize there was anything in it. Because I had found containers before, but they were empty.

DR. FISHMAN: It's just striking to me, because it sounds like for years he's been bailed out. Every time he gets into trouble he's been bailed out.

FATHER: That may be, but I. . . .

DR. FISHMAN: Don't talk to me, answer your wife. Talk to your wife about that, because it sounds to me like this is one more instance of bailing him out. But this time it could come out of your hide—the whole family's hide.

MOTHER *(addressing the therapist)*: I think I had mentioned it to him. He is not only in trouble, he has put us physically in jeopardy, too. Because we don't know when somebody's going to come and ransack our house. As a matter of fact, the other day, when one of his associates . . .

The parents' refusal to deal directly with each other is a pattern that needs to be challenged. I therefore attempt to get the couple to talk with each other.

DR. FISHMAN: Can I stop you for just a minute? Because I think you need to talk to your husband and I'm not sure he agrees. Because you agreed that you thought this was another instance of Carl getting bailed out.

MOTHER:	I said that?
CARL:	I'm not getting bailed out. You didn't bail me out when you told me I couldn't live at the house.
MOTHER:	Well, I think we keep extending the proverbial noose around your neck. You know, give you more rope for you to hang yourself. (*Addressing the therapist:*) I guess we just hope that there won't be a next time, or that he will change or something.
FATHER:	I guess that's what it amounts to, really.
MOTHER:	I have threatened to call the police. Unfortunately, I didn't. When he stole the money from me I should have. But I didn't.

I see here the misuse of hope. It was this pernicious hope that tomorrow things would be different that had kept the system from changing, even as the situation had grown more serious. Hope is part of what maintains the homeostasis. The job of the therapist is to create an enactment which vitiates the hope thus allowing new patterns to emerge that will result in change occurring right there in the treatment room.

Changing Reality Experientially

At this point in the therapy, I asked myself how I could create enough intensity to force the issue. How could I create a scenario that would no longer allow these parents to bail out their son and would also shake Carl's fundamental premise about himself? The object was to make Carl realize that he could not con his parents this time and to get the parents to see themselves as something other than willing pushovers. Perhaps the answer was to force the marital issue, to see whether the parents would pull together. If they could indeed support each other concerning the adolescent's misbehavior, the family would witness a moment of true transformation.

It was becoming apparent that these parents thought that talk could substitute for action. I decided to go for a complete and dramatic enactment, creating a crisis of trust between them.

MOTHER:	You are the son, I am the mother. You will do what I tell you, and if you don't want to, then you'll just have to be where you are. (*To Dr. Fishman:*) I keep saying the wrong things, I think.
DR. FISHMAN:	No, you keep saying the right things—more and more right things.

MOTHER: I have been saying that, but unfortunately, being a parent—I don't know whether you have children or not, but that's neither here nor there—you go the last mile with them, you know. And that's what I've always done with him.

DR. FISHMAN: Do you still have the vial? You know, I had a crazy thought . . .

MOTHER: What's that?

DR. FISHMAN: I wonder if he has anything with him right now.

MOTHER: He probably—I shouldn't say that—but unfortunately, my trust in him is nil, nil, totally nil.

DR. FISHMAN: Why don't you ask him?

MOTHER: Because he will lie.

DR. FISHMAN: Why don't you ask him?

MOTHER (*to Carl*): Do you have anything with you now?

CARL: No.

FATHER: Do you have any cocaine?

CARL: I don't have any cocaine with me now.

FATHER: Do you have any other kind of drugs with you?

CARL: No drugs, Dad.

DR. FISHMAN: Do you trust him? Do you believe him?

MOTHER: No. I don't believe anything he says anymore.

DR. FISHMAN: I think you should think about it. In other words, you should probably search him right now. And if he has anything, you can call the police—if you really want to give him something, to use your words, to go the last mile.

CARL: There's no way you're going to search me in front of a camera with people watching. You want to search me and go to that trouble, we can go in the next room and you can check me there.

MOTHER: What does it matter, Carl?

Many family therapists believe that by changing the family's reality the family's behavior will automatically change. It is essential, however, not just to create a new reality but to create it in the therapy room, so that a changed experience follows from the new reality. Thus, changing reality is only the first step.

The intervention practiced here changes the family's reality in an experiential way, so that new behaviors emerge focused around a specific problem. In this case the problem was whether or not to search the delinquent son. If the parents did not search Carl, especially after saying that this time they would be willing to call the police, they would reveal themselves as liars to themselves as well as to the therapy team. Moreover, they would have lied to their son about their resolve to stop his delinquency. On the other hand, if they did search their son they would be forced to change their pattern of accommodating to him—especially if they found drugs.

In the next segment we see the patterns change as the parents pull together and the family's reality begins to transform. As the parents respond to the challenge given them, new behaviors emerge and the family's notion of what is possible expands. Seeing that they can change gives the parents a renewed—this time legitimate—hope. More important, they realize that their son can change. They open up new possibilities from the multifaceted self and illustrate a lesson in complementarity. The parents realize, perhaps for the first time, that if *they* change they provide a context that demands a complementary change in their son.

CARL: You want to frisk me, we go in the next room, that's my final line. You want to frisk me, go in the next room.

MOTHER: I don't understand, what does it matter whether it's in . . .

CARL: Maybe a little pride I have left to myself while sitting here, you know.

MOTHER: I'm glad to hear you have some pride; I was beginning to wonder whether you had any at all.

CARL: You want to frisk me, we'll go right now into the next room.

MOTHER: Isn't it ridiculous that I have to do this.

FATHER: But if you have nothing with you why do you even object?

CARL: Because it makes me look like a fool, sitting there while you people frisk me. You want to frisk me we'll go in the next room.

MOTHER: No, we won't frisk you, just give me the jacket. I won't touch you at all.

CARL: We'll go in the next room and do this. You're not going to touch me in here. I mean that.

MOTHER: You see, you're upsetting me.

CARL: Well you're pushing me in a corner.

MOTHER: That's right, I am. You're right, I am pushing you in the corner. And who got himself in the corner? You or me?

CARL: And who's going to get himself out of the corner? That's why I left home, where I have to have you stand in the way of getting myself out of this corner.

MOTHER: You left home, so I am not in the way.

CARL: I'm better than I was a week and a half ago.

DR. FISHMAN: So, the question is, did he just lie to you?

CARL: Who knows? Let's go next door and find out. Me and Dad. Let's go right now and maybe we can find out if I'm right or not.

MOTHER: No, I know where all the zippers are, Dad doesn't. He's not as thorough as I am. I look behind pictures and find things.

FATHER: What's wrong with giving me your jacket, and I'll look at it here and now.

MOTHER: We won't have to touch your body.

CARL: What's wrong with going next door?

FATHER: Why not do it here?

CARL: Because I don't want to.

FATHER: Why not? Carl, give me your jacket.

CARL: Dad, I don't see why we have to do this.

MOTHER: He has a tendency to run.

When the mother says, "He has a tendency to run," I wonder if she is giving instructions to Carl—and if she is introducing a threat to her husband and me, hinting that if we increase the intensity and push Carl further, he will walk out.

FATHER: Because the more you object, the more that we believe that you've still got something, that's why.

CARL: Well, we can go next door and you can find out that I don't, okay? We can sit here fighting about it for the next hour. If you want to do that?

FATHER: I guess the next step we could do—I could maybe call the police.

CARL: They are not going to do it in front of a camera and ten people either.

FATHER: I don't want to fight you. Maybe if I call the police and ask them to go through your coat.

CARL: You're not going to do it in front of the camera and in front of six people. I'm not going to be a little freak show.

FATHER: You don't think that would be a freak show? That if the police came . . .

CARL:	No! I just won't allow you to go through my stuff. If you want to, okay—me and you, we'll look through my stuff. Me and you—family—not any of these other people.
FATHER:	I think it's gotten past family, though, Carl.
CARL:	No, it hasn't. You've gotten past family, and I haven't.
FATHER:	The "past family" is that the little secret has gotten to be about twenty-five or twenty-eight people. Do you know that?
CARL:	Who cares.
FATHER:	You don't care? So what's the secret?
CARL:	There's no secret. It's just. . . . Why let even more people know?
FATHER:	What's the matter? We might as well let everyone know.
MOTHER:	The entire neighborhood knows our business now.
CARL:	Considering you told every. . . .
DR. FISHMAN:	This is just distraction. You are accommodating to him and accommodating to him. He's saying right now, "Accommodate to me," and you, as parents, have to decide.
MOTHER:	Let me ask you this—what are we going to do, physically take it from him?
DR. FISHMAN:	What you have to do, whatever you have to do.

As I increase the intensity, I see the homeostatic pattern reemerging. The dysfunctional parental unit accommodates to Carl, but they also flip-flop.

MOTHER:	But I don't know what that is. He's (*indicating the father*) not physical. He's never laid a hand on him in sixteen years.
CARL (*to his mother*):	He wants to check my jacket, we'll compromise—you know, we'll go back there, and he can check my jacket.
FATHER:	No, I want to do it here, Carl. Please give me your jacket; please do it here.
MOTHER:	Take it off.
FATHER:	Come on, Carl.
MOTHER:	Not on your body, just take it off.
FATHER:	Carl, do it here. Come on.
CARL:	No.
MOTHER:	See, he has much more patience than I do. I could not do that. I would have to be physical. If it had been a girl. . . .
FATHER:	Come on, Carl. Please give me the coat.

I interpret the father's coaxing behavior as being in many ways homeostatic. His language suggests inappropriate closeness with his son. Here is a man talking to his sixteen-year-old son, who has just stolen from his wife and is selling cocaine on the streets, and he says, 'Please give me the jacket.' Figuratively speaking, he is the one who is "slipping fives" to his son. The mother's statement that she can be much tougher suggests to me that she has more distance. The goal at this point is to get the father involved and cooperating with his wife in creating an executive unit that is distanced from the son.

CARL: How about making it a little interesting for me, Dad. What's the benefit for me?

FATHER: The benefit is you're going to have a clean slate.

MOTHER: The benefit is some of your credibility might come back. If we find something—I mean, right now, as I said, I don't believe anything you say. I'm sorry but . . .

CARL: You don't believe when I say we're going to have to go next door and do this?

FATHER: That's not the point, Carl. The point is if you don't have anything, prove it.

CARL: I don't have to prove anything. I don't feel I need to prove anything.

DR. FISHMAN: Carl, why don't we step out so that you can feel free to do whatever you want.

MOTHER: Whatever that is I don't know. . . .

CARL: We'll go outside and you can check my jacket, if you really want to.

The therapist and I left the room to watch from behind the mirror, because we sensed that the intensity of the situation was being inhibited by our presence. Furthermore, the search was in many ways a private, difficult moment for the family. It was an intrusion into Carl's space, but one he brought on himself by violating his family's safety and personal property. The therapists did not want to do anything to inhibit these very polite parents. At stake here was the father's changing premise about himself. He was in the process of transforming his self-image from "I can be fooled" to "I will not be fooled." Carl, in turn, was shifting from "I can handle them" to "They can handle me."

The father stood up and Carl took off his jacket. The father went across the room to take it from him and opened the pockets of the jacket while the mother looked on.

CARL:	I couldn't even see some of those pockets.
MOTHER:	I don't even think you're funny, Carl. What about your [pant] pockets?
FATHER:	Turn your pockets inside out.
CARL:	There's nothing there.
FATHER:	Just prove it, that's all. Turn your pockets inside out.
CARL:	No, I'm serious, you guys stop now. I'm really serious. I'll go right out that door in a minute . . .

(*The mother stands up, crosses the room, and leans over Carl.*)

MOTHER:	Don't threaten me. Please don't threaten me. I said don't threaten me.
CARL:	I just did.
MOTHER:	I don't particularly appreciate that at all. You're a big man because you can threaten me?
CARL (*sarcastically*):	That's really good, Mom.
MOTHER (*her face close to Carl's and her finger pointing at him*):	Yeah, I know, it's very good—and you're ticked, right?
FATHER:	Pull out your pockets, Carl. Come on, stand up. Stand up, please.
CARL:	Dad, I'm really serious. If you ask me to stand up, Dad, I won't do it. You can check the pockets, I'm going to put this jacket on, and I'm going to walk out that door. I mean it.
FATHER:	Is that what you're going to do?
CARL:	Exactly.
MOTHER:	Carl, where are you going?
CARL:	I'm leaving. This is ridiculous.
MOTHER:	Stop.
FATHER:	Stop. Sit down there, please.
CARL:	You're making an ass out of me.
FATHER:	No I'm not. You did it to yourself.

CARL: No.

FATHER: You did it to yourself. Sit down.

(The therapist and I return, the search has ended, and nothing was found.)

CARL: Dad, I told you. If you wanted to check me, I was leaving. Did I tell you that, did I tell you that?

FATHER: And I told you a lot of things. Now sit down please.

CARL: You're both going to regret doing this. You know that don't you. You think you . . .

MOTHER: We're going to regret it? We have regretted so many things, Carl. Don't threaten me any more.

FATHER: That's the problem, Carl. The problem is you've brought all this on yourself. You've told us things that haven't been the truth before.

CARL: Well do I get an apology then for all this?

MOTHER: Wait a minute, how many things have *you* apologized for?

CARL: You guys didn't believe me that there was nothing in my coat. Now, do I get an apology?

FATHER: Do you apologize to us? No, come on.

MOTHER: How many times have you lied to us? Do we get apologies for all those?

CARL: Yes you do.

DR. FISHMAN: Also, what happens the next time?

FATHER: The next time it will be the police, there's no doubt about that. I'm not fooling around any more.

CARL: I guess I can't come home then till all my debts are paid off.

DR. FISHMAN: Should he come home, if he's not going to school? If he were going to school, it would be important for him to be at home. But if he is not studying. . . .

> Not using drugs, coming home and returning to school are the issues around which the organization of this system has to change. The parents need to decide whether or not they want the child to reintegrate into the family.

The question at this point is how to maintain the intensity. The parents had successfully pulled together and created a parental subsystem by searching their son. What content could be used next to maintain this new, inchoate pattern?

In treating adolescents, the therapist must be alert to the adolescent's extraordinary skill in outmaneuvering adults and destroying the source of authority. Carl's threat that he will not come home if his parents are tough with him is just such a maneuver. I turned his threat around, however, insisting instead that Carl can come home *only* when he begins acting appropriately. In situations like this the therapist must move quickly to keep the adolescent from taking away the parents' instrumentation—their tools for harnessing their son. Before the threat becomes too open and the parents begin to get scared, the therapist must prevent the adolescent from asserting control. The parents must remain in authority and retain their sense of dignity: they, not the adolescent, must remain in control of the door.

While acting to keep the parents in control, however, the therapist must be careful not to slam the door on the delinquent. The goal with this family was to set up a situation that would allow Carl to come home under certain conditions, one that would allow him to regain his position as a rightful member of the system if he lived by the rules: to come home he must go to school; to come home he must not use drugs. There was no hope of Carl becoming a "good son" again if his parents did not act like parents. Once this was accomplished, we could focus on ways for Carl to redeem himself in the system. Our purpose is not merely to put the parents back in charge, but to put them in charge in such a way that they encourage their son to earn his return to the family.

In the sequence that follows I try to sponsor a moment in which the parents uphold their power and, at the same time, the adolescent is provided a road back. Other objectives are to give the adolescent the opportunity to learn that he can challenge the rules without destroying the source of authority and to allow him a chance to make amends. By providing a way for amends to be made, the therapist also encourages the process of atonement.

FATHER:	Well, he's not going to come home and cause the problems he's had for us recently. There's no way.
DR. FISHMAN:	I've heard that. But how many times have you heard that?
MOTHER:	We have not discussed it amongst us, but there's no way that he's going to keep his money as such. He doesn't know this yet, but. . . .
CARL:	I know that, but all you said. . . .
DR. FISHMAN:	All right. Why don't you talk together about that. Would you want him to come home? If he wanted to go to school, it would make sense for him to be at home. Most sixteen-year-old kids are in school.

CARL: Can they make you leave before you're eighteen? Can they kick me out of the house? Legally?

Suddenly this adolescent, who has been threatening to hurt his parents by leaving for good, is not about to leave so easily. Power has been restored to the parents and the adolescent is testing its extent. He wants to keep his nest—and misuse it. At this point the therapist must encourage the parents in their position of newly won control and rightful indignation.

MOTHER: Wait a minute. Let's not talk about legalities, because your buns should have been gone a long time ago—and not to any country club.

DR. FISHMAN: So talk about that. I don't know that he should come home. From what I've heard you're always accommodating to him. What you just did here I think is very important and exactly what he needs. I mean, if he were to go to school or work, there would be something. But the fact is he's on welfare.

Who accommodates to whom is an important issue for this family. If the parents continued to accommodate to their son, his behavior would not change. Only changes in the boy's context would force different, more functional sides of the adolescent's self to be expressed. Later he could be allowed the freedom to choose functional behaviors needed to be a member of this system. What should be negotiated here is the price of membership in the family.

CARL: The fact is they don't want me back in school right now.
FATHER: Yeah, but that's your doing. Not ours.
MOTHER: That's beside the point. I mean, I don't know if he could do anything positive right now, because he doesn't get transportation.

The father has gotten tough, but once again the system reverts to the flip-flop undercutting of its own authority. By switching and saying that the boy has no alternatives, in effect the mother bails him out. The therapist must act to short-circuit this threatened return to accommodation.

FATHER:	That's his problem.
MOTHER:	I know it's his problem.
DR. FISHMAN:	Maybe you should take a taxi.
CARL:	They don't have any taxis.
DR. FISHMAN:	See, that's just an excuse.
CARL:	That's not an excuse. If I had a way. Last time I went I hitchhiked. They made me stop—I had to quit my job at the gas station.
DR. FISHMAN:	No. That's just an excuse.
CARL:	But it isn't.
DR. FISHMAN:	But does he believe that you will not let him come back?
MOTHER:	He has told me I will. When he gets ticked at me he says, "You know, Ma, I know you'll let me come back." He actually told me that. (*Turning to Carl:*) The last time you were home.
DR. FISHMAN (*to Carl*):	You're probably right. If they found cocaine on you, do you think they would call the police?
CARL:	When?
DR. FISHMAN:	Ever.
CARL:	After a while. They probably will, yeah.
DR. FISHMAN:	When you're forty-five and living at home?

I deliberately exaggerate to convey to the parents that they have heard all of this before.

CARL:	I don't know. I really don't know.
DR. FISHMAN:	That's what I think.
MOTHER:	Excuse me, Doctor, but I was a chaperone at the high school dance. (*To Carl:*) Tell him what I did to you.
CARL:	You tell them.
MOTHER:	I beg your pardon—I'm asking you to.
CARL:	I don't remember.
MOTHER:	You don't remember—come on. I was a chaperone. Smoking was supposed to be prohibited, and I caught my own son. I warned him once, I warned him the second time. The third time I took him—I tried to take him—to the principal's office. He ran. The whole school knew about it.
DR. FISHMAN:	Did anything happen to you?
CARL:	I had to stay after school.

DR. FISHMAN: I think you're right, Carl. They will never—you'll be living there probably when you're forty-five. Do you have a nice home?

MOTHER: Um-hm.

DR. FISHMAN: Good. (*To Carl:*) Not bad. (*To parents:*) You see, I think the key to really helping him is to only let him move back if he's back in school. If he cuts school again, he leaves.

FATHER: Well, his next alternative—he's been kicked out of this school twice.

DR. FISHMAN: I don't want to talk about the specific schools, because we don't have much time, and I wonder if the two of you could make up your mind regarding that. You see, I think one of the tragedies of his life is that you didn't call the police yesterday.

MOTHER: Well, as I said, when I found it I thought it was empty. Wouldn't that be silly if I had called the police and said, "Here's an empty packet"?

DR. FISHMAN: Of cocaine? Yes, they would know what he used it for.

MOTHER: I know that. But I mean I didn't know if there was anything in it.

DR. FISHMAN: Your wife is just defending him.

FATHER: Um-hm.

MOTHER: No. I'm defending myself, because I didn't open it. You mean to say I could have called the police and they would have done something for an empty packet?

DR. FISHMAN: Ask your husband, he's the expert.

FATHER: I don't know. I'm not an expert in coke, I. . . .

DR. FISHMAN: The question is, this is his whole life. What happened yesterday is his whole life. In other words, he was—again—accommodated to. He didn't have the consequences of his actions. I think you have to make a decision right away—to decide that you don't want him back.

MOTHER: I have threatened so many times—as I said, I . . .

DR. FISHMAN: He doesn't respect you at all.

MOTHER: No.

DR. FISHMAN: He thinks you're idiots.

MOTHER: What do you mean?

DR. FISHMAN: He steals from you. He thinks you're idiots.

FATHER: I think what you have said—as far as school—because we feel one of the most important things is his missing school and he doesn't seem to think so.

DR. FISHMAN: He doesn't have to. He's so comfortable.

FATHER: Without it, yes. He has no problems because he doesn't have to go to school.

DR. FISHMAN: That's right. So talk to your wife. We only have a few minutes.

FATHER: I think that probably ought to be the criteria then.

People only become competent when their childish narcissism, which tells them they will always be taken care of, is challenged and broken. In this family the adolescent's narcissism is still strong. He has never worried about his future because he has never really had to address serious life problems. The therapeutic goal here is to provide an existential crisis for this young man, to drive home the realization that he is responsible for his own life and that if he is to make anything of his life he must rely solely on his own efforts.

DR. FISHMAN: You just got an invitation.

CARL: When I go back to school—which isn't for a year, at least.

DR. FISHMAN: You'll find something.

CARL: There's no school that will take me.

DR. FISHMAN *(to the parents)*:   See, I think this is a terrible tragedy. You can't change him at all—but you can change yourselves.

FATHER: In what respect?

MOTHER: To not coddle.

DR. FISHMAN: Not coddle. Not make excuses for him. You can do nothing directly for him. But for the two of you, you could be a team and you could absolutely make it very clear that he doesn't come home—probably ever again. That doesn't mean you can't talk to him, whatever.

MOTHER: Well, that's what I said. I said, live somewhere and come visit me on weekends—we can have a beautiful relationship, but I can't live with him.

DR. FISHMAN: You really want that?

MOTHER: He could visit.

DR. FISHMAN: I would hope not every weekend.

MOTHER: No, I say visit. You know, like—like maybe you do, you go see your mom on weekends?

(Later in the session Carl left the room and I spoke with the parents alone.)

DR. FISHMAN: You know what's fascinating? Each one of you vacillates. First you're soft, then your wife's soft.

MOTHER: Well, that's right—as I said, I have my strong days and I have my weak days.

DR. FISHMAN: That's why you need each other so much.

MOTHER: I have always been the bad guy. It is sometimes very hard to get some support from him to be the bad guy. Because I guess I feel more strict. I don't know, we just think differently in so far as child raising is concerned.

DR. FISHMAN: Well, what are you going to do now?

MOTHER: Are you saying we're never supposed to leave him in the house again? I don't want him living with me, but certainly I want him to come visit me.

DR. FISHMAN: Ask your husband.

FATHER: That's fine. If he wants to visit. But no more staying—he's done, he's gone.

DR. FISHMAN: You're saying that now.

FATHER: I'm saying that now, and I'm meaning it now.

MOTHER: And I'm saying that now. Until he calls crying one night—which he will do.

FATHER: But no, that's the time you can't continue to give in to him. Because if you give in to him that time, you've lost. I'm better off if I have time to sit down and think about it a little bit. Not that I'm going to come up with any better answer, but I don't react spontaneously.

MOTHER: And I'm just the opposite—I'll be spontaneous.

FATHER: It's like the doctor says, if you think about what the possibilities will be ahead of time, and then try and plan for them. . . .

MOTHER: Know your next step—always one step . . .

FATHER: Try to keep two steps ahead of him, and . . .

DR. FISHMAN: You know, I have another solution. All you have to do is call your husband first before you make any decision. And vice versa.

What I am trying to do is dispel the myth that separate strength is the answer.

Many parents believe that toughening up individually will be enough to improve the situation, but in fact they could each be strong individuals and still produce a delinquent child. The truth is that the delinquency is abetted by their tendency to make decisions independently of one another. The real answer is for the parents to close ranks and be strong as a couple.

THE FOLLOW-UP

By the end of this family's therapy the parents were together, though perhaps not as wholeheartedly as I might have hoped. In such situations, however, change is often slow, and this family continued to struggle. When they returned home the parents were able to stick to their agreement and insist that their son not come home until he agreed to the changes. At first Carl moved in with his grandfather and was able to recruit him as a new homeostatic maintainer for his delinquency. However, the grandfather died and Carl went back to school and returned home. Subsequent problems in the family shifted away from Carl and centered on his older brother's heavy drinking, which in fact became the focus of later follow-up sessions.

In retrospect, the therapy was a success in that it reinforced the parents as executive authorities and nurturers and resulted in Carl's eventually returning home and ceasing his delinquent behavior. In truth the family system was only partially transformed. The therapy would have been more effective if it had included both the grandfather and the brother. In this case the therapy should have continued until *all* members of the system—not just Carl—were stabilized.

I was a consultant in this case. Had I been the primary therapist I would have seen to it that the therapy addressed the larger context. In Carl's case it apparently was not essential, probably because his talent for school, once he began applying himself, provided a nondelinquent context that confirmed him. But his brother needed some work with the broader context to find a nonfamily situation in which he could be competent. This would have been essential in helping him leave a family that seemed to need at least one problematic child. When the children had finally left, then, the parents would have been able to work out their problems directly. The follow-up session described in chapter 11 demonstrates this powerful point.

Summary

It is important to remember that family therapy is not the art of keeping families together. The focus of family therapy is on understanding family processes in order to know what needs to be done to create a more functional system. In the case of delinquency it is especially important to move quickly to change behavior, even if this means separating family members. If the adolescent is allowed to persist in his dysfunctional behavior and senses that he can get away with it, the delinquency will become more and more impenetrable to therapeutic efforts.

In treating delinquency it is essential to work with the full context of the adolescent, which of course includes peers. At times it might be effective for the therapist to see the delinquent with one or two peers. Even more important, however, is the necessity of encouraging the parents to become acquainted and, if possible, develop a friendly relationship with the peers. If this external context is positive, it needs to be encouraged as much as possible. If it is negative, an attempt must be made to remove the adolescent from the pack. And then the hard job of therapy—the job of creating the "unwolf-like wolf"—begins.

Claude Brown, author of *Manchild in the Promised Land* and a graduate of the Wiltwyck School for Boys, describes what was for him the transition point, when he first thought he might not spend the rest of his life as a petty thief in Harlem, stealing and fighting and maybe getting killed. He tells of a work assignment with a woman who saw his potential and told him that he had intelligence, that he "could be somebody." Eventually she gave him books to read, biographies of such people as Jackie Robinson, Albert Einstein, and Albert Schweitzer. He read the books and eventually asked for more, reaching a point at which "Cats would come up and say, 'Brown, what you readin?' and I'd just say, 'Man, git the fuck on away from me, and don't bother me'" (Brown 1965, 157).

As I understand, Brown's escape from the delinquent world was by finding competence in another, socially enabling context. Suddenly, as he saw other lives in the biographies, he saw alterative scenarios for his own life. As he became engrossed in the world of books, he developed the skills to succeed and to escape from the poverty that bred the delinquency.

4

The Runaway Adolescent: A Therapy of Options

Wedn'sday morning at five o'clock as the day begins
Silently closing her bedroom door
Leaving the note that she hoped would say more
She goes downstairs to the kitchen clutching her handkerchief
Quietly turning the backdoor key
stepping outside she is free

She (we gave her most of our lives) is leaving
(sacrificed most of our lives) Home (We gave her everything
money could buy)
She's leaving home after living alone for so many years
Something inside that was always denied for so many years—
She's leaving home
Bye-bye
—JOHN LENNON and PAUL McCARTNEY

THERE WAS A TIME in our history when running away from home might have been seen more as an adventurous passage of adolescence rather than as an admission of family problems and failure. Children longed to go off with the circus or dreamed of floating down a river with Huck Finn. The paths taken might not have been easy, but in the end the adolescent returned to loving relatives and assumed more responsible, adult behavior.

Such is the stuff of romance and literature. As Blair Justice and David

F. Duncan (1976) point out in their perceptive article on runaways, these fantasies of the past pale in comparison to today's harsh realities. They quote from a report by former senator Birch Bayh:

Unlike Mark Twain's era, running away today is a phenomenon of our cities. Most runaways are young, inexperienced suburban kids who run away to major urban areas . . . they often become the easy victims of street gangs, drug pushers and hardened criminals. Without adequate food or shelter, they are prey to a whole range of medical ills from upper respiratory infection to venereal disease (Bayh 1973).

In the decade and a half since Bayh's report, the problem has only worsened. Lappin and Covelman (1985) report estimates of five hundred thousand to two million runaways per year—approximately one out of every seven teenagers. Other figures confirm that as many as a million teenagers run away from American homes each year (Young et al. 1983; Farber et al. 1984). Most of these adolescents continue to come from white suburbs. At least half are female, and many are no older than thirteen or fourteen. As researcher Helm Stierlin (1973) points out, "Only drug abuse, with which it has many links, rivals running away in importance as a mental health issue for young Americans. And, like drug abuse, running away taxes your abilities for understanding and treatment" (p. 56).

There are, of course, many speculations about the causes of this epidemic of runaways. What research has been done seems to indicate that the families of runaways experience more breaks and stressful life events such as death, divorce, and separation. In addition, runaways are frequently subjected to beatings, problems of alcoholic parents, recurring arguments between separated or divorced parents, and the negative experiences of a father's prolonged unemployment (Roberts 1982). Obviously such family experiences are not uncommon. It is now estimated that for noninstitutionalized adolescents in the twelve to seventeen age group, 10 percent of boys and 8.7 percent of girls run away from home at least once (Farber et al. 1984). These are children who leave or stay away from home on purpose, knowing they will be missed, and who intend to stay away for some time.

How are we, as family therapists, to approach this problem? Perhaps we should begin by keeping in mind the basic fact that for many adolescents running away is a final weaning from a difficult family organization; in fact, in many cases running away is the best of few good alternatives, some of which could lead to self-destructive behavior through drugs or suicide. This chapter takes a look at such an adolescent—one who *chooses* to live on the streets because her family was, in her view, unsupportive.

The middle- or even upper-class teenager who runs away may not be so different from the child of poverty who lives in the streets: they both perceive their homes as lacking in basic nurturing and support. For these children, the chaos of the home seems unrelenting, while the chaos of the streets can at least be offset by anonymity and the companionship of peers in like circumstances. To adults running away seems radical and foolhardy; from the adolescent's viewpoint, however, in addition to escape it can offer the realization of a universal quest for freedom and independence.

Often a runaway adolescent's most compelling complaint about home life is that it is "too strict." A look just under the surface, however, usually reveals that the problem is not a frustrating strictness but a parental conflict triangulating the child. It is common in these families for one or even both parents to be going through a mid-life crisis. For example, career change, caring for members of the older generation, and marital conflict may all be increasing the vulnerability of the family system. These developmental crises in the adult subsystem frequently stimulate behavior problems in the children. Unfortunately, it is often the case that the parents then focus exclusively on their adolescent's behavior, neglecting to address their own problems which in part were responsible for their child's difficulty. Thus we have the makings of a vicious circle.

In working with such families therapists should attempt to distinguish the parental and the adolescent's issues. The object is to keep the parents in their executive position in the family hierarchy while enabling them to present *options* for the child. If parents misunderstand the therapist and think the solution is only a matter of getting tough, the therapy will be futile. The therapeutic goal is to help the parents both to be firm and to provide options.

General Principles

CREATING A THERAPY OF OPTIONS

The runaway child sees no other option but to run away and escape. In these rigid, inflexible family systems there is a paucity of alternatives which can be effectively expanded through a therapy of alternatives, a therapy of negotiation. The ultimate goal is to establish a family system in

which the child does not have to run away from home but can *walk* away
from home at the appropriate time. This therapy should end when options
are opened not only for the child but for the parents as well, options that
enable them to come to terms with the developmental issues stressing the
family system.

HELPING THE ADULTS NEGOTIATE BETWEEN THEMSELVES

The first stage in the therapy of families with an adolescent runaway
is to help the adults learn to negotiate between themselves in the presence
of the children. This negotiation should serve to distinguish parental and
adolescent issues as well as to prepare the parents to begin negotiating
with their children. In this type of family system retrieval of the child is
most likely to go awry when preparations for the adolescent's return *pre-
cede* the ability of the parents to negotiate between themselves. When this
happens the adolescent may return home, but the environment of the
home may demonstrate the same chaos that caused the child to leave in
the first place. And even if the adolescent does not run away again, other
forms of rebellion are likely.

In order to facilitate the process of family negotiation, the therapist
must first deal with the unrealistic fears on both sides that are keeping the
system stuck. The fear of what the adolescent might do keeps the parents
incapacitated and renders them ineffective. The fear of parental actions
frustrates or frightens the adolescent and drives him to run away. A principal task for the therapist is the acknowledgment and handling of these
fears. Frequently the parents have great difficulty in assessing and handling their own fears. Unrealistic fears may indicate doubts in one or both
parents about their own adequacy and safety within the family. The therapist must face this issue directly and early in the course of treatment, for
the distortion of fears and the resulting confusion about what is or is not
likely to happen may put the adolescent in real jeopardy. For example, in
the family about to be discussed the father was terrified that if he asserted
executive authority over his daughter she would rebel further and perhaps
become a prostitute. The mother was fearful of her daughter holding a
grudge against her for years to come.

WORKING TOWARD THE ADOLESCENT'S PARTICIPATION IN THE
TRANSFORMATION

Of course, the adolescent has fears as well, and these must also be
addressed if the process of negotiation is to be successful. Every effort must
be made to get the adolescent to participate and to believe that a negotiated

transformation of the system will open real options and alleviate fears. This participation needs to begin in the treatment room and then be extended outside to the family context.

Ultimately, the prognosis for permanent change in families with adolescent runaways depends on the parents' capacity to be both firm and flexible. Their foremost responsibility is to keep their children free from harm, but this can never be accomplished if the adolescents themselves are not given the opportunity to be free. To the extent that the therapist can help parents retain their executive power while allowing their children real choices, the therapy will be successful.

Clinical Example:
Maria, On Her Own at Age Fifteen

Our illustrative case revolves around Maria, the fifteen-year-old daughter of a prominent family and the third of five children. Her sisters were nine, twelve, and seventeen years old. Her brother was twenty. At the time of the therapy Maria had moved in with a boy in a poor area of the city and had been living apart from the family for some months. What precipitated Maria's leaving home was her categorical refusal to follow her parents' rules.

ASSESSMENT USING THE FOUR-DIMENSIONAL MODEL

History

The family was well established in New Jersey. The father was seen as a very successful professional. The parents had met at a European high school and had been married for twenty-one years. Their family backgrounds were very different. The mother's family was Latin and quite emotional, whereas the father's English family was more distant. The father had been seeing a psychiatrist because of problems at work and was taking antidepressants at the time of the family therapy.

Development

Maria's father had been extremely depressed over the last nine months. He worked as a highly successful graphic designer in a very competitive advertising agency, and he feared that he might be losing his ability to handle the required technical details. The mother had been confronted with the developmental pressure of having her children need her less and less as they became increasingly autonomous. Trained in anthropology to the bachelor's degree level, she did not feel that she had any immediate employment opportunities.

Structure

The parents had an extremely distant relationship. I learned in the course of the therapy that their sex life had been essentially nonexistent for at least two years. Each of their relationships with the children differed drastically. In this family the mother was the more concerned parent, while the father was initially intimidated by the girl's threats. As the mother became braver, the father became increasingly subject to the girl's intimidation. The symptomatic child had a special position in the family: not only was she the child who most challenged the rules of the system, but she was also a strikingly beautiful girl. With her dark beauty she reminded one of the very young Elizabeth Taylor in *National Velvet*.

Process

In this intellectual, educated family, there was a firm belief that all difficulties needed only to be explained away. However, there was no negotiation per se, just intellectualization. The girl moved out when the parents told her that if she didn't follow the rules, she would have to go. There was no precedent of the family as a laboratory in which to practice negotiation skills; this was partly the result of the extreme terror this family had for any emergence of conflict.

The effect of a system like this on the therapist is very interesting. It is easy to become seduced by the high-level talk and to feel as though one is conversing with one's college professor. On a social level this family could be friends with the therapist, and this presents a real challenge: the therapist's job, after all, is to transform the system, not to be a good guest at a cocktail party. The therapist should act as a foreign body in the system, making the system challenge its rules and obliging it to change.

THE HOMEOSTATIC MAINTAINER

When the parents were challenged in the session, first one and then the other would act as the homeostatic maintainer. The father acknowledged the necessity for negotiation but actually excluded his wife from the process. At an early point in the therapy he undermined attempts to have the parents come to an agreement by trying to convince the therapist that he should see Maria alone. As the session continued I attempted to have the father function as a co-therapist to convince his wife to join with him in bringing their daughter home. The mother would demur from supporting her husband and insisted that the daughter should be involved in the decision. I found myself having to constantly monitor whichever parent was carrying the baton in order to address the therapy toward neutralizing the homeostatic efforts.

WORKING FOR BRIEF THERAPY

In my experience the key patterns enumerated earlier lead to fast change (see page 20). By dealing with the parental dyad prior to bringing the child home and then working with the system to create a therapy of negotiation, the likelihood was increased that the return would not be short lived.

THE THERAPY

Searching for a Therapeutic Middle Ground

With this type of family system the adolescent can be very confused as to what is allowable behavior and what is not. The parents vary between rigid enforcement and extreme indulgence. These were not really tough parents; they were parents who resorted to a choking, tough response after having allowed their daughter too much leeway to do whatever she wished. Maria experienced her parents as giving permission and then taking it back, and she interpreted their ambivalence as betrayal. Therapy had to be directed toward making them less indulgent and more thoughtful about a variety of issues. They would then not appear so rigid when the time came to make demands.

What appeared on the surface to be a rigid family system was in reality a system in flux. The system remained unstable because it had no mid-range, no effective modulation. Since the parents could not work out a sense of balance for themselves or for their marriage, they could not respond to the needs of the adolescent. What Maria needed was not extremes but a gradual development of autonomy.

In families with runaways, we assume that the adolescent is not running away because he or she is crazy. Rather, the adolescent is running away because there is something very poisonous in the family context. The goal of therapy, then, is to help create a different kind of context, one from which the child will not have to escape. Thus, in this case, close attention was placed on *what Maria had to run back to.* She could not run back to a family that would only become more authoritarian. It had to be a family that had learned compromise and found a middle ground. It had to be more executive, yes, but also more balanced, without the discordant equivocation between the parents that frustrated the girl and caused her to seek escape.

I speculated earlier about the contextual pressures that were keeping the parents rigid and pushing them to act in extremes. The father was blocked in his work and having a profound mid-life crisis. The mother was undergoing a vocational reentry crisis; and this mutual upheaval was causing a deep dissatisfaction with each other as spouses. The parents could not be flexible, either with each other or with their daughter; they remained wrapped up in their own lives and problems. Because of the constricting pressure of their individual life crises, dialogue had ceased— and dialogue, as we know, is part of what permits the family to be a flexible organization. With this family, then, the system had become rigid as the parents acted to maintain it by focusing more and more on their rebellious daughter, thus diffusing their own difficulties. Of course, their difficulties with Maria exacerbated their sense of helplessness in their own lives.

The parents in this family were no longer a couple, but merely two individuals in crisis. Their marital evolution had stopped as each spouse withdrew into him- or herself. The adolescent's acting up was the only thing that brought them together; in this sense, her running away can be seen as constructive. The job of the therapist was to help rework the system so that the parents would have more than their troublesome daughter holding them together.

Reworking the System

All family systems are idiosyncratic because of the discrete personalities of the participants. An important ubiquitous therapeutic drama for the therapist to consider, however, is: the reorganization of the system so that there is a functional structure for all family members to differentiate by the imposition of boundaries in a way that is gradual and life-enhancing rather than abrupt and pathologically arresting. The underlying issues can often be addressed through negotiation, leading to the shifting of the homeostatic maintainers for increased freedom and openness.

As we have seen, in the therapy of the runaway adolescent we are most often dealing with a rigid system that must be opened up through an emphasis on negotiation and the creation of options. Obviously this therapeutic task can be accomplished only by getting the family to deal in a more functional way with the runaway. But before a family can learn functional negotiation, it is first necessary to reorganize the system so that the parents speak with a single voice in challenging their adolescent. In this case, the parents did not really know what they wanted from their daughter, so they worked against each other. They seemed to take turns overprotecting the girl, alternating in their firm and lax reactions to her running away. The therapy had to focus on getting the parents to act in concert and then on creating coherent generational boundaries within the family. Afterward, the reentry process had to be closely monitored so that as the family healed, the individual space would be reworked and the adolescent could exist within the system instead of feeling she had to find space through extraordinary means.

In the session that follows, the overriding emphasis was on establishing negotiation—negotiation within limits, but negotiation nevertheless. These parents experienced themselves as being frequently incapable of exercising firm executive functions, such as establishing curfews or rules against certain behavior. This action was perceived as "against our nature," a violation of the very concept of who they were as people and as a family. But to preserve themselves as a family this had to change. The parents had to learn to negotiate between themselves and with their daughter. They could not assume that the "expert" would mediate their problems for them.

The following excerpts are all from the second therapy session.

DR. FISHMAN:	Did you have a chance to talk, just the two of you, without the participation of the kids? Because it seems to me that you are really in a fix.
MOTHER:	What do you mean?
DR. FISHMAN:	Well, I'm not sure what you are going to do.
MOTHER:	Well, I can't help but think there must be other methods.
DR. FISHMAN:	Talk together about that and see if you can get an idea.
MOTHER:	We do so much (*she laughs*). Now we come to talk to you.
DR. FISHMAN:	Well, talk together about it. I have really told you the way I see it. The way I see it, you have to choose a way to present a united front to your daughter. There is no other alternative. So talk together about it.
MOTHER:	Well, just let me say okay, then, if you say we have to choose that we want to negotiate. But you seem . . .
DR. FISHMAN:	Check with your husband, and see what he wants.

FATHER: Yes, I also feel that we should negotiate, for the simple reason that I feel that we don't know each other well enough, so to say. I think we would find out much more about what Maria really wants.

In these few minutes the rigidity of the family could be perceived. The mother was inflexible in her effort to transform the problem into a dialogue with the therapist, which compelled me to handle her inexorability with a dismissal. Realizing that her request was a red herring, a distraction, I centered her back on her husband. That was precisely what she did not want to do. She wanted to talk about negotiation, but she did not really want to negotiate. Instead she wanted to engage me in a useless battle. The rigidity was expressed in her inability to turn to her husband for an exchange. The counter to that, 'the therapeutic management, was to rechannel her firmly back to her task.

DR. FISHMAN: What Maria wants? She's only fifteen. I'm not so concerned about what Maria wants. She is in a dangerous situation!

FATHER: Well, I am. I'm telling you what I think. You asked me to say something, so give me a chance to say it. I have been very interested in knowing what Maria really wants. I think that's the way to get to her. Not in a session or a whole group, but probably the best way, so that she would be able to open up more, would be if she had a session with you alone. And then, after that, you two would be able to come to a formulation that she would be willing to tell us about, as to what her aims are and her ideas. And then we may be able to talk about that. I think right now she is sort of pushed into a corner and as a result of it she takes a very extreme position that she wants to do exactly what she wants to do, and there is no giving in on anything. Which is a very good negotiating position, let's face it.

When an impasse develops over the process of the adolescent's reentry into the family, the therapist often finds that the problem is a misperception by one of the participants. In this case, the father perceives negotiation to be a process that should exist between one adult and the child. He expresses more interest in his daughter than in his wife as a way of avoiding conflict with his spouse. In such a situation the therapist must refocus the parents so that it becomes clear that at this moment the issue is not the negotiation with the girl but negotiation with each other, whatever the risk of conflict. In this first stage they must decide between themselves what they want, then negotiate for it with the girl. Confusion about this sequence of negotiation can paralyze the therapy.

DR. FISHMAN:	Maria, how long have you known the person you are living with?
MARIA:	Maybe a month.
DR. FISHMAN:	A month?
MARIA:	Three weeks, something like that.
DR. FISHMAN *(to the father)*:	Your fifteen-year-old daughter is living with a—how old is this fellow?
MARIA:	About eighteen.
DR. FISHMAN:	An eighteen-year-old man. And you're talking about getting to know her better! So that, right now, she is in a good position to negotiate. I don't understand.
FATHER:	She lives with this fellow. She lived with a family before. And she's trying to come out.
DR. FISHMAN:	But she's only fifteen.
FATHER:	I know she's fifteen.
MOTHER:	I guess what you are saying—can one force her? One can physically force someone to do something and that will work to a certain point. But can you change their being, their essence?
DR. FISHMAN:	That will happen later. But right now, if you wanted her home by 9:30 when she lives with you, because you worry where she is. . . . Now you don't know where she is at all. What can you do? How can you stay away?
FATHER:	We are not happy about it.
DR. FISHMAN:	But how can you tolerate it—as a father?

The father is the homeostatic maintainer at this point. To disrupt the homeostasis, I challenge him by telling him he is accepting the unacceptable.

FATHER:	All I can say is that if she is home I feel that what she is doing is things that I don't approve of, but at least I can live with.

It was necessary to point out to these parents that they are not being as decent and protective as they believe—that they are wrong in acting as though the problem will resolve itself if they simply wait their daughter out. The goal of the therapist is not simply to provoke the parents into getting tough, but to change the homeostatic mechanism that is keeping this system stuck in its unhappiness.

We also see here that the family pathology did express itself in a way that was immediately detectable. The father did recognize the necessity of negotiating with his daughter, but he also acted to exclude his wife from the process. If this exclusion were allowed to continue, it would only reinforce the homeostasis and doom the negotiation. As a result I had to interrupt and start the sequence afresh. The therapeutic operation had to be directed to restoring the parents as a working hierarchy of caretakers in agreement. Only then could they begin to successfully negotiate their daughter's return to the family in the proper role of a girl requiring supervision.

Creating Intensity

In the next sequence, the therapist struggles against the rigidity of the family system, increasing the intensity in order to overcome the system's persistent conflict avoidance.

FATHER: If she is so insistent on living away, that is just incompatible. Then, in a sense, to a certain extent, at least temporarily, I have to wash my hands of it.

DR. FISHMAN: I understand that. That's how you've been thinking. But how can you stand it?

FATHER: Well, partly by not thinking about it too terribly much. Because I have enough problems to worry about as it is. Not because I love it, or because I think it's great. But because it's very, very undesirable—one of a number of undesirable occurrences.

MOTHER: We saw no other solution, except that Maria would leave home.

DR. FISHMAN: Do you worry about her? How about at 11:00? Do you worry about her?

FATHER: Not too often, my friend.

DR. FISHMAN: Do you ever wake up in the middle of the night?

FATHER: Seldom. I do occasionally, but not very often.

DR. FISHMAN: Do you ever wake up early in the morning?

FATHER: I think that some days I don't think about her at all. Maybe that's wrong, but it's true.

DR. FISHMAN: But the days that you do think about her. Do you worry and wonder where she is?

FATHER: I hope she's at work. I hope she's sufficiently tired from work that she'll go home and go to bed, as I think that many days she does.

DR. FISHMAN: This fellow that she's living with, do you know anything about him?

FATHER: No. But I think it's better that she's here than if she runs off to San Francisco and becomes a prostitute. Which may very well be a result of what you're suggesting.

DR. FISHMAN: I'm suggesting she become a prostitute?

FATHER: No, you're not suggesting it. I say what you are suggesting might lead to it. If we try to restrain her physically, the first thing she'll do—not go to school so we can catch her. Next thing she'll do is—so the cops can't catch her—go to New York, or New Orleans, or San Francisco, Tijuana, Mexico or someplace, and make a living the way she can. The quickest and easiest way is to become a prostitute. I think that's far worse than what she is doing now.

Changing Realities to Challenge the Homeostasis

At this point in the therapy it became clear that the parents' conflict avoidance had to be directly challenged. Only then would husband and wife begin dealing with each other, which was the first step they had to take before they could effectively deal with their daughter. My way of encouraging this transformation was to shake the homeostatic maintainer. In taking this approach, however, the therapist must be prepared for some counterattacks. In this case the father reacted by implying that I endorsed a dangerous means of control that would lead the girl to worse problems, such as prostitution. These concerns were, I believe, not valid; the girl had never raised the subject of prostitution nor made any threats along those lines. I saw the father's preoccupation with such fantasies as his way of maintaining the homeostasis, in the sense that these fears kept him from addressing the conflictual issues at hand: the necessity of joining with his wife and bringing his daughter home. It was just such fears on the part of the parents that allowed the girl to prevail, because their fears prevented them from taking a decisive position on their daughter's behavior. The father was afraid that any attempt to control the girl's behavior would cause her to reject her parents and assume the even more negative identity of a prostitute. As a result they chose to do nothing. However, I believe the situation was in reality quite different. It was not firm action but the lack of it that was pushing their daughter to extremes.

This case cannot be explained satisfactorily without considering the complexities and the contradictions of the family system. It is not that these parents were unconcerned for their daughter's welfare; their overconcern with the danger their daughter was in was helping to maintain the unwanted behavior. The therapy had to work to make them aware of the *real* danger rather than the imagined one. Moreover, these parents, who felt extremely guilty and afraid of losing their child, at the same time saw their daughter as grown-up and beyond their reach. They saw the girl as a sophisticated, urbane, very sexual creature—a view that I challenged. The system's perception of the girl was full of contradictions; she was both an ultrasophisticate and a child. These contradictions helped to produce the madly oscillating system from which the adolescent felt she must flee.

DR. FISHMAN: Do you agree that your daughter could become a prostitute? Could you see if your wife thinks that?

MOTHER: I would like to think that Maria has more—basically that wouldn't happen. But I cannot give myself any kind of guarantee that it wouldn't. And that's what I'm afraid of.

FATHER: Maria is so hard in her aims—and so resistant.

MOTHER: At least now we have communication with her, and at least we are talking to each other. I think that's worth something.

FATHER: I think that's very true, what you say. At least if we try to get back together again, we will not first have to find out who has to say the first word. Because at least we are talking a little bit. Not much, but by God, it's going to take a long time for that to happen. And it's that state we have.

DR. FISHMAN: So the two of you are not satisfied.

MOTHER: No, we're not.

FATHER: Not "satisfied"—that's the wrong word.

DR. FISHMAN: Well, you say you want to negotiate and you say you can't . . .

FATHER: I didn't say that.

DR. FISHMAN: . . . at this point.

I am slowly moving the parents to accept the fact that they have to begin to negotiate right now, with the daughter in

the room. However, to do this, the father's objection that
the daughter cannot negotiate must be overcome. This
requires tenacity and intensity; if I give in to the father's
understanding of the situation, nothing will change.

In the following segment, exasperated, I urge the father to negotiate, and the girl, like the archetypal adolescent, makes her plea for freedom, decision, and choice. He cannot succeed without his wife.

FATHER: At this point. Not today, right? I said we should find out more closely what it is Maria really wants.

DR. FISHMAN: Why don't you ask her.

FATHER: I said, I don't think it will come out. I will ask her if you want me to, but I don't think it's going to come out in this kind of conversation.

DR. FISHMAN: Go ahead. Maria, could you tell us in any way?

FATHER: What are really the most important things that you feel that you want, and you cannot have at home?

MARIA: I can say it pretty generally—a lot more freedom. I mean, I could say a lot of little things. Like, if I wanted to stay somewhere for dinner. I would have to call, and a lot of times you'd say no. And I wouldn't see any reason why I couldn't. That's little things. Or maybe more of your acceptance of what I want to do. Not so much you guys just thinking, well, we're the parents. I know that's the way it is, you guys are the parents, and you make the rules. And I have to listen to them and go by them, or I can't stay in the house. I don't really know. Just being able to make more of my own decisions, even if they're not right. So I'll find out if they're not right. But I don't want you to have to tell me how I can run my life, who my friends should be, who my friends shouldn't be, and where I should go. I guess that's part of it, at least.

Working with the family of a runaway can be very tricky. While participants may speak as if they want to negotiate, what they may really want is recognition as the "good" negotiator. They want to be seen as acting in accordance with the goals of the therapist, but this does not necessarily mean they want to achieve those goals. In this case the father wants to be the good guy, the one who does the negotiations, as opposed to his wife, who is excluded. If permitted, the father would negotiate everything with the adolescent as though his wife were not present. But in fact he is not in favor of true negotiations; rather, he is attempting to prevent the girl from feeling pressured. This is his way of expressing his special bond with his lovely daughter and seeking never to lose her favor.

At every moment of hesitation I continued to try to get the parents to talk, and to convey to them the message that *they* had to change in order for their daughter to come back.

DR. FISHMAN: These are things that will haunt you for the rest of your life. If she's out on the streets and she gets hurt, this will haunt the two of you for the rest of your lives.

MARIA: But I can get hurt anywhere.

DR. FISHMAN: Talk together about how you are going to change your wife. You need to change her, so that your daughter will come back.

FATHER: I don't think she wants to be changed.

MOTHER: Locking you up for the next six months is not precisely living at home.

> *Predictably, the father defends the girl, persisting in his attempt to ally with his daughter. While the father is developing this alliance, the mother simply expresses disagreement. At this point, she begins to act as the homeostatic maintainer. And when I try to get the father to deal directly with his wife, he resists and again acts to maintain the homeostasis. Here is a process in which the role of homeostatic maintainer shifts back and forth between husband and wife, an illusive process that ultimately stymies change.*

Later in the session Maria leaves the room and I continue the task of getting the parents to be of one mind. To dissipate the fears each has of exerting executive authority over their daughter, I attempt to unbalance the system by supporting each parent as they challenge the other. This gentle intensity confirms each parent while challenging their reality that their daughter is a potential powderkeg.

DR. FISHMAN: Are you going to bring her home tonight or not?

MOTHER: I feel more courageous now because I simply feel that there's no other choice. Because I don't think we can say that much more. I mean, the kids can have their say. We pretty well know about Maria, but the other kids, they talk to us. So we pretty well know what their ideas are.

FATHER: It's good this way. When Billy was a baby and he would start to cry for no reason at all, I could stop him, essentially by punishing him by spanking him very lightly. And he would cry a little louder and a little louder, and then he would stop. And I remember I tried the same with Cathy. She would just get louder and louder and I realized that she would die from loss of breath before she would give up crying. So, it's certainly a point that I realized that a certain form of punishment certainly didn't work with her. And in effect, with Cathy, nothing would work and she's been very loud and very noisy about it. Maria, so far nothing's worked except she's been very quiet about it. She doesn't say anything—keeps to herself, does what she wants. . . .

MOTHER: You mean you really feel that Maria—well, I think she does want to come home. I've heard that often enough from her, and from others, but . . .

DR. FISHMAN: You need to decide—the two of you. You are having a terrible time coming to this decision. You need to decide.

FATHER: I find so many—I can't go back to the present state.

MOTHER: We're afraid. Okay, I'm afraid. I'm afraid to take such a big risk.

FATHER: Maria has very much the attitude that what happens to other people won't happen to her.

DR. FISHMAN: You're taking that attitude. You're saying that she is not going to get murdered in that neighborhood.

FATHER: She also feels this. For example, we saw this movie of a girl who ran away from home, became a prostitute, came home again, ran away again. She was watching with us, and I'm sure she felt, "That's not me."

DR. FISHMAN: It's a big decision, but you need to make it.

MOTHER: Is this what you recommend to most of your families that fall into the same category with us? It scares the living daylights out of the kids. And then they come back and, you know—they get together, get with it again. I mean, if it works that magically, then I think it must be wonderful.

FATHER: I think it would be magical if we would get to the nitty gritty of this. It would be pretty raw.

DR. FISHMAN: That's right. And then you're in charge. And then she's relieved, because she's not so powerful. But talk together, because I don't hear the two of you getting even close.

FATHER: I feel like she is under an awful lot of pressure right now, and I don't think we (*indicating himself and his wife*) should add to it.

MOTHER: I also feel that if we should not say, well, next Friday you have to be home, I think that would be wrong.

FATHER: But do you feel that you could try this and stick to it? Because let's face it, when we walked up here we believed not a single word of this whole thing. And so, are we just being talked into it by a clever car salesman, or do you actually feel that it may work?

The parents are attempting to escape, via the therapist, from the unavoidable task of having to negotiate as two grownups in charge of their runaway daughter. Notice that it is not the husband who demands they get firmer, it is the therapist. I handle their objections not by engaging in a debate, but by responding with silence and then returning to the task. Fortunately, the husband had already been sufficiently pushed on the issue and was ready to consider negotiating with his wife. The following sequence shows the exchange of fears and the beginning of real negotiation.

MOTHER: I guess I was hoping there would be another solution—a different solution.

FATHER: I feel the same way there. (*He pauses*) Yes, that's about the way my father ran the family and I did have some bad moments; although I must say I still do respect him. (*Quietly, to his wife*) So, shall we?

MOTHER: (*Sighing and smiling to herself*) We took the risk when we asked. We said she could leave, so she left, and we (*glancing at husband*) took that risk.

FATHER: You've got to stop being nice to her when she's hurting.

MOTHER: I know.

FATHER: You don't have to stop being nice to her when she's good.

> *A real dialogue is beginning between husband and wife. They glance and look at one another, almost as if they were a young couple flirting. It looks like a genuine process, and that produces a moment of great reassurance for the wife when the husband says, "You don't have to stop being nice to her."*

DR. FISHMAN: That's an important distinction. That's a very important distinction.

MOTHER: Maybe I should have. I've never stopped being nice to her. That's the trouble maybe. I've always tried to be. . . .

DR. FISHMAN: You need to be with him. Do you want to get her?

(Maria reenters the room and the negotiation with her continues, this time with the parents united as a negotiating team.)

FATHER: Okay, so we need to talk about it a little more. I don't think we've said anything very new. And if so, we haven't tried to say anything behind your back. But we have decided that you are coming home tonight. We will help you pick up your stuff.

MARIA: I don't have any stuff to pick up. Some of it is at Sally's house.

FATHER: Do you need it tonight?

MARIA: No.

FATHER: Okay, then you can just come into the house.

MARIA: What's that for? Just tonight?

FATHER: No. To stay.

MARIA: And what if I don't?

FATHER: Do you want all the rules—what if, and what if—so you will know exactly how far we will go? You have to realize we are your parents and we are in charge.

MARIA: Well, I didn't come to this . . . (*She begins to cry*) I didn't come to these meetings to be told that I have to come home. You said we'd come here to compromise. I mean, I didn't have to come to these things. I don't think it's really fair to me to tell me I have to come home, when you told me before if I wanted to live . . . You sort of told me I had to leave if I didn't want to go by the rules. So I chose to do that, and we agreed that I could do that. And that's what I've been doing.

FATHER: And you also agreed to come here for help. And apparently the form of the help is that you are to come home, Maria. It's not that we are trying to play a mean trick on you. But we have become convinced that the only way to take care of you properly is that you come home.

MARIA: So, I walk right out the door then.

FATHER: I don't want you to. And I don't think you're going to. There are other things that we can try, but I hope you won't try.

MARIA: I don't think doing this is very fair, and I don't think it's going to help anything. You guys can tell me that I have to come home now, and live at home—and you also told me to leave. I've been doing all this stuff on my own. I just found another place to stay.

The father tries to justify and defend the impossible position they had worked themselves into by having told their daughter to leave.

FATHER: We didn't tell you to leave. We told you at home there were certain rules, and if you couldn't live with them, that you would have to leave. That's what we said, okay.

As Maria pushes and negotiates for her right to more autonomy she seeks an admission from him that her particular perception was a reasonable outcome of the way she had been treated. Now the father has to retreat, by saying, "We didn't tell you to leave." He equivocates—a process that always exacerbates problems between parents and adolescents.

MARIA: And we agreed that I could leave and I did leave. And now you're telling me I have to come home. After you just told me I should leave.

Maria immediately reacts and goes after the essence of the confrontation: their waffling behavior.

If the adolescent is not validated in her reading of reality, she will find it impossible to go back into a family context that nullifies her process of independent thinking and perception.

The father now shifts and abandons his rigidity.

FATHER: It's also changed for me. It's not something that I come to very easily. But I realize by letting you go, we have not been taking care of you as parents should. We have changed our minds. It's not to be mean to you. You might say you've had a vacation. I hope it was good for you— was good for us—but things can't continue like that.

The father's formulation could, of course, be construed as just going soft again. But in the context of the negotiation, this exchange reflects the father's readiness to concede that his daughter can perceive reality correctly. It shows that he is sensitive to her perceptions. Prognostically this is a very good sign. This beginning of sensitivity will encourage the girl to return without feeling that she is going back into hell.

DR. FISHMAN: *(to the mother)*: Why don't you say something? Because Maria needs to know where you stand.

MOTHER: I agree with Daddy. I think it's been a very hard decision for us, but it doesn't look at this point as if there's any other way. And while you have been living away from us, it hasn't been because we wished it, and thought that was the solution. It was a temporary solution, because we saw no other way at that time. Things were at a point where we just didn't know what else to do. In the meantime, we have come here for help. Time has passed. We've seen some things that have happened to you, the life that you are living—the life we are living—and we feel it's time for you to come home. Do you know that we've always been afraid of things that can happen to you? You are under age. You can be picked up and you can be taken advantage of. There are a lot of things. You have been slipping in your schoolwork—late many times. And I give you a lot of credit for the things you've done, but there are also things that . . . .

FATHER: She has been able to take care of herself—she has. But that doesn't mean walking the streets alone at night.

MARIA: How do you know that? Where do I walk alone? I barely ever walk alone. I was just talking to Cathy about that. If I lived at home that could happen to me anyway.

FATHER: No, because we don't let Cathy walk alone by herself at night. We always walk her back to the dorm, or something. None of us goes out at night alone by ourselves.

MARIA: I don't walk alone anywhere.

MOTHER: Well, that's not the most important thing. I would hope in some time you will find other friends, other activities, something that will be more meaningful in your life.

MARIA: You've been saying that to me for two years now. I'm not going to change my friends, and I don't want to change my friends. You can't make me do that.

DR. FISHMAN: That's true. Your parents can't make you change.

> *Seeing that both mother and daughter are about to get into an impossible hole, I try to validate the girl's position and relieve the parents. While aligning myself squarely with the parents in applying pressure on the girl, I had to be ready to jump over to her side when needed.*

The fact that the daughter fought the parents to the end was a very healthy sign. Although she was going back home, the protest was extremely important. When runaways simply capitulate, one must wonder what they will do next.

The therapy with this family moved to a new stage as the parents learned to amplify their daughter's freedom, so that being home did not justify her fear that she was returning to a prison. I predicted to the parents that at some point their daughter would test them. Indeed, shortly after her return home, she stayed out overnight. She was punished for this offense, and in the ensuing crisis the parents showed that they had learned much about the art of negotiation. A follow-up one year later revealed that Maria did not attempt to live away from home again until she left for college in Chicago—one thousand three hundred miles away—with the blessing of her parents.

Summary

In the course of the therapy these parents had become empowered. When their daughter came home she challenged her parents, but the system withstood the challenge and the girl stayed home until the end of high school. The therapy continued to focus on the family as a caring place where the children had limits and a voice, a place where they could negotiate.

A number of subsequent sessions with the parents addressed their problems of distance from each other. The father stopped his individual therapy and the medication. Eventually the couple became involved in starting a business together.

5

Treating the Violent Family: First Do No Harm

> Yet each man kills the thing he loves,
> By each let this be heard,
> Some do it with a bitter look,
> Some with a flattering word, . . .
>
> —OSCAR WILDE

FAMILY VIOLENCE is generally thought of as physical abuse or the threat of physical abuse between family members. The exact prevalence is not easy to determine because the phenomenon is often narrowly defined and because statistical data is often based on disparate sources such as emergency room reports, police statistics, or self-report. Nonetheless, ample evidence exists, as Richard Gelles writes, for "exploding the myth that family violence is infrequent or rare" (Gelles 1980, 878). Surveying a nationally representative sample, Murray Straus, Richard Gelles, and Suzanne Steinmetz (1980) found an incidence of physical violence between marital partners of 16 percent in a one-year period and 28 percent over the course of the marriage. Gelles (1980) reports estimates of child abuse from six thousand to one million incidents annually, and David and

Patricia Mrazek (1985) state that more than two thousand child mortalities per year occur as the result of physical abuse. As Peter Jaffe and his associates (1986) point out, increased media attention highlighting the problems of family violence has lead to a growing public awareness of the need for specialized services, such as shelters for battered women and child advocacy groups.

The most common explanation for the persistence of the phenomenon in our society is that each generation learns to be violent by being a member of a violent family (Straus, Gelles, and Steinmetz 1980). Researchers have also consistently found that family stress and a lack of warmth and sensitivity within the present family are factors that contribute to the perpetuation of violence (Gelles 1980; Carroll 1977; Mrazek and Mrazek 1985).

For the clinician I believe the most important factor is the presence of stressful family relationships in the *present* context. In his 1977 study of the transmission of family violence between generations, Joseph Carroll found that even among those who had been abused as children, less violence was associated with those experiencing a high degree of marital happiness. Reporting on factors contributing to child abuse, Mrazek amd Mrazek (1985) point out that a primary factor in triggering abuse is stress within the family as well as in the surrounding community. It is these contemporary forces that unleash the violent expression and therefore must be addressed directly in therapy.

It is often the case with violent families that those who commit violence see themselves as victims rather than as abusers. As Salvador Minuchin notes in his *Family Kaleidoscope* (1984), perpetrators of family violence often see themselves as helplessly responding to the victim's baiting and plead for understanding of their plight as a "helpless victimizer."

It is my contention that the plight of both victimizer and victim in violent families is actually a problem of invaded boundaries. In fact, violence in families is usually precipitated by an intrusion of boundaries, an intrusion that leads to helplessness, fear, anger, and confusion, and ultimately to violent expression. In dealing with violent families the therapy is directed toward making or strengthening boundaries—toward reorganizing the family rules around established, functional boundaries. If the family can create a functional boundary in the therapy room, there is greater assurance that they will be able to do so outside the therapy room. The questions the therapist must pose begin with these: How is the context within which these family members operate making them helpless? What maintains the problem? What is the cause of the extraordinary stress that has pushed the system to the point that violence emerges?

General Principles

Working with explosive, violent families requires the therapist to keep firmly in mind four basic principles: first do no harm; create a therapy of experience; develop positive regard between family members; and deal with both the family and the broader context.

PRIMO NO NOCERE

The first principle should be every therapist's primary concern: *primo no nocere,* "first do no harm." The great physiologist Walter Cannon coined the concept of the wisdom of the body to explain the homeostatic mechanisms of the human organism. The therapist must assume a similar stance when working with families, even those with very serious problems. There is a kind of wisdom of the family, in that the system's organization, problematic though it may be, does serve some function and should not be summarily dismissed. The do-no-harm principle is especially valid when dealing with violent families, and the therapist must tread carefully when reinforcing the adult subsystem. To do otherwise may jeopardize the safety of a family member.

This makes working with such a system especially difficult, for in order to move forward the therapist might have to issue directives that could undermine a participant's protection. For example, in the case that follows, there is a dysfunctional coalition between mother and son against the father that needs to be lanced. But there are also moments when the mother needs to recruit the son for help against the father. Thus the therapist must be vigilant and monitor the situation closely, so that the therapy does not vitiate a life-saving coalition. Indeed, this is the special dilemma of the therapist treating a system that has violence. For the therapist could unwittingly deactivate an apparently dysfunctional system that is, in fact, exquisitely functional on some level.

A THERAPY OF EXPERIENCE

An important concept that we borrow from the logicians is that one cannot prove a negative. One cannot prove that violence will not recur. Because the therapist is in the vulnerable position of deactivating a possibly life-saving coalition, it is essential to have reliable criteria for progress. In other words, the therapy must be one of *experience*. After all, if we are in good conscience to say, "Mother, give up your protection," then we must also be able to assess and change the dysfunctional patterns then and there in the therapy room as they emerge in family enactments. Moreover, the therapist must work to change these patterns quickly, because the family is involved in a potentially dangerous situation.

As mentioned in chapter 2 there are a number of characteristic patterns that can be seen and transformed in the therapy room. The cross-generational coalition mentioned earlier is one such pattern. Once identified, such coalitions are addressed, split, and broken down so that restructuring can occur right there in the therapy room. Another common pattern is conflict diffusion by activation of a third party. Here the therapist must address the system's ability to resolve conflicts between dyads, especially between mother and father, without involving a third person as a means to defuse the tension. Complementary or symmetrical schizmogenesis is another pattern often encountered in violent families. In these systems patterns of mutual escalation must be disrupted in order for family members to begin building more functional interactions.

Since we cannot prove a negative—that the violence will not recur—the therapist must take extra care to verify the existence of new functional transactions in the treatment room. In the absence of such new behaviors, or if the old patterns reassert themselves, then the therapist must take appropriate action to assure the safety of family members.

WORKING TOWARD POSITIVE REGARD BETWEEN FAMILY MEMBERS

As stated earlier, the therapy deals initially with breaking down coalitions and establishing a more functional hierarchy, with the therapist watching vigilantly to see that new patterns are indeed emerging and that the system has not been destabilized to the point where real danger exists. When functional patterns do begin to emerge in the therapy room, the therapist can be reasonably sure that the danger has passed. One of the key functional patterns to foster, then, is the development of positive regard between family members. This pattern needs to be sponsored and reinforced in the therapy room.

Joseph Carroll (1977) found that mediating factors for transgenerational violence included a high degree of physical punishment that modeled violent behavior, combined with either a lack of warmth or a high degree of stress within the family. Thus therapy must work to create a context where there is more warmth and less stress. Of course, the diminishing of violent punishment goes hand in hand with changes in other areas.

As demonstrated in the clinical case that follows, in working with violent families the therapist must deal with and reverse the prevailing degradation. Clearly, a kind of degradation can be felt by both victim and victimizer. The therapy needs to address feelings of self-worth and foster an atmosphere of respect so that more positive sides of the self can emerge. One important way of handling the degradation felt in such situations is by enabling a process of negotiation to take place from positions of mutual respect.

Therapy with violent families must deal not only with the system's organization and structure but also with the affective tinge that colors a relationship. Without addressing the basic issue of *liking or disliking*, we will not change the violent adolescent, and therapy should not be concluded until positive regard has been established.

DEALING WITH BOTH THE FAMILY AND THE BROADER CONTEXT

William Goode (1971), in his resource theory of intrafamily violence, states that the more resources a person can command, the less likely it is that he or she will actually deploy violence. This theory, which is supported by empirical data (O'Brien 1971; Gelles 1974), concludes that violence is a last resort when other resources have failed or are lacking. The most difficult ecological forces are those involving the family's larger context, such as poverty. For situations such as these the therapist must function like a traditional social worker to help the family deal more effectively with available resources. David and Patricia Mrazek (1985) report that families that are unable to use community resources are more vulnerable to stress and therefore are at a greater risk of resorting to violence.

It is essential that the therapist not delay the process of dealing with the broader context. Because the pattern of family violence can become readily entrenched and is so difficult to undo, any potential contributing factor must be addressed quickly. Those people and forces destabilizing the system must be included—for example, the extended family, estranged or divorced spouses, or helping services that may be working at cross purposes. With violent families, the dangerously explosive behavior involved requires that the inclusion (or the planned *ex*clusion) of these forces must begin immediately. For example, part of the problem in the context of the clinical family in this chapter was that each parent's individual therapist was acting, unknowingly, to stress the system. It became necessary, therefore, to ask the couple to either discontinue their individual therapies or bring their therapists into the family sessions.

In this family, I believe the father's alcohol usage is a problem. In the true contextual point of view, it is a pattern that emerges as secondary to the severe stress within the system. And the effective stabilization of the father's drinking problem could be achieved by working intensively to transform this stress in the family. In the event that the problem had not abated, I would have tapped the broader context and suggested adjunctive treatment modalities such as AA. This would strengthen the context and serve to stabilize the father in a non-alcoholic mode.

Clinical Example: Mike, His Mother's Gladiator

In this family not only were the children violent but the parents were as well; they were two sides of the same coin. Violence was pervasive in this family and was essential to the maintenance of the dysfunctional homeostasis.

The family lived in New Jersey and had arrived in therapy because the oldest boy, Mike, was in danger of losing his scholarship at a private school. The parents were in their early thirties. The father was employed as a clerk in a retail store while attending night school to complete college, and the mother was a full-time nursing student who worked evenings as a waitress. There were four children: Mike, age fifteen, Thomas, fourteen, Vanessa, eleven, and Cindy, ten.

Father was a weekend drinker who frequently drank heavily on Friday nights and would come home drunk. At such times he would often hit his wife, and a physical battle would ensue between them. When this occurred the older boys, particularly Mike, would often attempt to rescue their mother by entering the fight. The boys had rageful fantasies about their father. In fact, Mike had gone so far as to threaten to kill him. This was a family in which tempers were short and fists likely to be thrown at any provocation.

Both parents were in individual therapy, but there had been no coordination of their separate therapies—neither had seen the other's therapist and there had been no joint sessions. These individual therapists, knowing only one side of the problem, gave advice out of context which served to compound the spouses' mutual anger and exacerbate an already explosive situation. For example, Mother's therapist told her to "go to your husband

and tell him what you feel." But at home, when she tried to get a hearing she was only further frustrated and became hopelessly demoralized, feeling that she had no voice and no power.

The mother was preparing for her own career but saw her plans in jeopardy because she and her husband had not effectively completed the job of child rearing. The two eldest boys were each enduring a difficult adolescence. Mike had run away from home and was failing in school, and Thomas had been tormented by desires to be violent with his father. The family members were constantly involved in one another's business and offended one another in explosive ways; they had great difficulty with maintaining boundaries and with not hurting one another. Each experienced a sense of entrapment. The system offered restricted choices for all. The only way to go with this family was to attempt a radical weaning of the parents from the children. The outstanding goal was to disengage the parents from the kids and establish functional boundaries.

ASSESSMENT USING THE FOUR-DIMENSIONAL MODEL

History

This family was in great upheaval and in a repetitive pattern. The father would go out and get drunk and violence would emerge, followed by a period of rapprochement, when the father would become extremely contrite. It was apparent that these parents, who had married very young and never finished their own childhoods, were trying to complete their growing up now. They were extremely sensitive to educational failures in their children because they had dropped out of school themselves as a result of adolescent rebelliousness.

Development

Clearly, the developmental pressures were extreme in this family. Three of their children were adolescent, the eldest fifteen years old when therapy began. The parents were aged thirty-four and thirty-two. But it was apparent that these adults were, in a way, addressing their own adolescent needs by seeking continued education in order to better themselves.

Structure

The father and mother had many marital difficulties and had been separated for eight months, reuniting a few months before the inception of therapy. They were not only distant but embattled; there was a war be-tween them—and it was by no means a cold war.

Because of his drinking and his consistently angry and critical role, the father was overtly estranged from his children but also very intrusive and overinvolved. The mother and children were much closer.

Other structural factors to be considered included work conditions, financial difficulties, and pressures on both parents due to their own con-tinued schooling: they were, after all, raising four still-needy children while addressing jobs and difficult educational ventures.

Process

In the therapy room there was an almost palpable sense of tense-ness and anger among the family members. Everyone monitored one another—especially the father—very carefully. They seemed to fear that the father would suddenly blow up. It was interesting to note that the observers watching this family from behind a one-way mirror also ex-pressed a fear of the father; there was even some speculation that he could be an "ax murderer."

As the process patterns emerged it became apparent that the family used a third person to diffuse conflict. The more impressive sequences were the symmetrical battles that flared up between the kids and, espe-cially, between the parents.

THE HOMEOSTATIC MAINTAINER

The mother served as the homeostatic maintainer, activating to smooth things over when tempers started to heat up and often joining with the oldest boy. This served both to diffuse the conflict and to protect the mother. It was essential to diffuse the tension, since the first priority was the safety of the family members. Unfortunately, the manner in which this was done—a coalition between the generations—ultimately led to greater tension and conflict.

THE THERAPY

I was the supervisor behind the one-way mirror. In the room were the therapist and the family: the mother, the father, and the four children, all casually dressed. As we started the second session, the therapist began to explore the issue of responsibility, challenging the family about who was in charge of what in the family and getting immediately to the issue of boundaries.

Dealing with responsibility is essential in treating adolescents. The three adolescents in this family had to undergo developmental estrangement, the realization that one is responsible only for oneself and that ultimately one's parents cannot rescue one from one's responsibilities. Indeed, adolescents who believe that parents can rescue them will not work diligently. In the following excerpt the therapist tries to facilitate the experience of developmental estrangement for Mike by examining the boundaries between the generations.

THERAPIST:	But, I mean, they know when you have to study, what you have to study.
MIKE:	I tell them when I have to study at home. I told Mom.
THERAPIST:	So you mean your studies are not *your* responsibility. They are not something that you handle on your own.
MIKE:	Handle on my own?
THERAPIST:	Yes.
MIKE:	Well, there was a particular thing the other night . . .
FATHER:	She's asking you the question in general and once again you're evading the facts.
MIKE:	No. I'm asking you then. . . . I told Mom I had to study for history, which I did a little at school.
FATHER:	Okay. But what the doctor asked you is, whose responsibility is it to study, yours or ours?

The father's mood seems to be related both to the son's pain and to the pressure brought by the authority of the supervisor behind the mirror.

MIKE:	I don't know. I really don't.
FATHER:	That was a simple, down to earth, good question.
MIKE:	I don't know. Last night you had done that, yes.
FATHER:	She asked you a general, general question. Nothing about last night. Nothing about last night. All she said to you was—and I will repeat myself again, okay—whose responsibility is it, ours or yours?
MIKE:	For me studying?
FATHER:	Yes.
MIKE:	Well, lately it has been yours.

FATHER: That's what she asked. But whose responsibility is it, is what she asked you.

Both father and son were increasingly angry in their responses. The mother looked exceedingly uncomfortable and pained. From my assessment of the family it was clear to me that the threat of violence and the fury expressed between Mike and his father could only be allowed and tolerated if the parents were split. The boy was his mother's protector against the father, and his mother supported him against the father. The boy was furious at his father for abusing the mother as well as for not respecting him. As for the father, he felt he would not be driven to drink so much if he did not feel that his family was against him.

As the father and son argued, the mother seemed increasingly tense, looking from one to the other. I saw her position as untenable, triangulated between these two people whom she loved very much. At this point I decide to intervene to try to transform this dysfunctional organization. It was keeping these people helpless by creating stress sufficient to cause the violation not only of interpersonal boundaries but also of the societal injunctions that say that violence, especially to loved ones, is a sin.

I enter the room as a co-therapist, my only goal at this point is to support the mother. This support, I believed, would add sufficient intensity to help this obviously tormented mother and wife out of her agonizing position. I sit next to the mother and start speaking to her softly. After introductions, I focus the family's attention on the question of responsibility.

DR. FISHMAN: You know, I think that is a key question. I agree with you. Whose responsibility is that?

FATHER: It's a simple question, also.

DR. FISHMAN: Yes, absolutely.

FATHER: This is what I go through at home with him. He does everything he can to avoid giving me a direct answer. (*To Mike:*) Don't you?

The threat of harshness or violence from the father is obvious and is read by Mike.

MIKE: No, but I don't know what you are going to do if I give you a direct answer.

FATHER: You usually say to me, "Dad, I hope you don't get angry, but may I speak," and I will say to you, "Yes, Mike". . . .

MIKE: Lately it's been my responsibility, okay.

FATHER:	Lately?
DR. FISHMAN (*to the mother*):	Are you comfortable with that, Patty?
MOTHER:	With Mike? I don't know.
FATHER:	With the answer.
MOTHER:	Oh, yeah, he's right.
FATHER:	I still think he's avoided the question.
DR. FISHMAN:	I'll tell you what occurs to me and what comes through the mirror. (*To each parent:*) It's that you work hard and you work hard, but you don't pull together. You pull in separate directions. Is that your sense?
MOTHER:	Yes.
DR. FISHMAN:	So it must be confusing for you, Mike. What do your folks want?
MIKE:	They expect me to have marks like I always used to have.
DR. FISHMAN:	You know, that happens. I'm telling you that I think it's a confusing message.
FATHER:	Okay, but may I ask something at this point? Michael has been told, and all the children have been told, that if they bring home a sixty, as long as I know—as long as we know that they tried their best, nothing will happen to them.
DR. FISHMAN:	Sure, but what do the two of you want in terms of whose responsibility it should be—his grades?
FATHER:	His.
MOTHER:	I want him to be responsible.
FATHER:	It's his school work, it should be his responsibility. It's the rest of his life, not ours.

Both parents are overinvolved with their children, blurring the boundaries within the system and subordinating the relationship between husband and wife. When one parent joins with the children, the other is left out in the cold. In the sequence that follows the father's overinvolvement is expressed in anger.

MIKE:	Well there is nothing I can say until I bring up my marks. I'm not going to try yet, but when I do—*when* I do—then I'm gonna have a lot to say.
FATHER:	You're losing me. I don't understand what you're trying to say.

MIKE: When my marks come up, when I have something to show for it—I'm going to have a lot to say.

FATHER: Can I ask you what you mean?

MIKE: Well, I mean, whatever you say will all have to be wiped out. You can't tell me that I'm stupid anymore. You can't tell me that I can't do nothing.

It is apparent that Mike puts up with his father's insults because he feels he is not justified in complaining as long as his poor school performance continues. Here he is saying, in effect, "Insult me once more, trespass boundaries and disrespect me once more, and I'll attack or leave." The vindictiveness and revenge felt by the boy are strikingly on the surface. It is becoming clear that this cycle of escalating degradation and boundary trespassing is what breeds violence.

FATHER: Mike, did I explain to you what I meant by the word *stupid*?

MIKE: Yes, but you can't say it anymore.

FATHER: I guess I won't be able to.

MIKE: You won't and I'll make sure of it.

FATHER: But then won't you feel better about it, too?

MIKE: I'll feel better because I'll be going out.

FATHER: Won't you feel better because your marks are higher?

MIKE: For me, yes. I'm not doing this for you.

FATHER: Well, hopefully, it's for yourself.

MIKE: It is for myself—and for Mom. Me and Mom.

As the system is being perturbed, the homeostatic mechanism emerges. The father's disparagement of Mike entrenches the boy deeply in a coalition with his mother. We see how the mother and the youngster are connected and overinvolved and how the father is left out in the cold. And to the extent that the father increasingly feels excluded, he is more likely to feel helpless, to feel that he has no allies in his own family. And, of course, the more isolated he feels, the more likely he is to drink and then become violent.

TOM: Why won't it be for Dad?

MIKE: Because it won't.

FATHER: Why won't it be for me?

MIKE: Because, Dad, you know something? I really don't really like you at all.

FATHER: Why?

MIKE: I just don't like you. You say I have a mean streak in me. Well, it shows in you more than it does in me.

In a sense Mike is right. And here the father is being paid with the same coin with which he treats his son: meanness.

FATHER: What brings the mean streak out?

MIKE: Probably me.

I lean over and speak softly to the mother, asking her how she feels when her son talks to her husband this way. She says, "It tears me apart. It's killing me." I urge the wife to support her husband rather than the youngsters in order to free them from the grip of triangulation. This is counter to her reaction in everyday life, where she normally sided with the children, not the father, thus allowing him to lose authority in their eyes. My purpose is to try to lance the coalition that is central to the maintenance of the violence in the system.

FATHER: Why does "you" bring it out?

MIKE: You know why, Dad. You ask me questions that—you know. You know.

FATHER: I want them to know.

Here we see the shaping of the violent adolescent. Of the many sides of his son's multifaceted self, the father picked the "rotten kid" to reveal. The father was trespassing boundaries and setting his son up with questions that show the boy in a bad light. The father's seemingly malevolent intent was to expose the boy and thus control him because the young man could be painted as always being wrong. But Mike saw through these techniques of entrapment and thus revealed his intense dislike of his father, responding with hurtful words: "I really don't like you."

The father, of course, is a victim of this triadic system as well. He goes into overkill trying to expose the rottenness of the boy because he feels overpowered by the coalition his wife and son have formed against him.

The father's violence to the young man is by now fundamentally established. The son *cannot* trust him and will do nothing for him, and the father is effectively out as an executive authority. The system is a breeding ground for the malevolent self to grow and to strengthen.

Since the homeostatic mechanism has emerged—the overinvolvement between mother and son—I can work toward fostering the emergence of new patterns right there in the room. "Do whatever you have to do so that your son doesn't talk to your husband this way," I say to the mother, fully aware that the son had felt justified and that the mother had felt compelled to support him.

In lancing the mother-son coalition, however, it was important to keep in mind the do-no-harm principle. The mother had actively communicated with the boy by gesture or position in a way that had recruited him. The therapist had to be careful, therefore, not to let the mother deactivate a support system that she needed. Unless there were radical changes that eliminated the mother's need for her son's protection, Mike would have to keep playing macho games with his father.

MOTHER: Mike, I don't want you talking to Dad like that. I don't like it. I don't like what I'm hearing.

MIKE: But the reason we were supposed to come to these sessions is to say what we feel.

MOTHER: All right. You are. But I don't like it. And I can say that, too—I don't like it.

MIKE: I'm sorry.

MOTHER: I don't like hearing you talk to him like that. I really don't.

Mike was caught in a situation where he had been called to the rescue, then told he was bad when he attempted the rescue. The therapist had to be especially attentive to the stresses in the transformation so that the family would allow the boy to feel competent and confirmed in other, more functional areas.

FATHER: Do you think I pick on you needlessly?

MIKE: No. But sometimes you do.

DR. FISHMAN
(*pointing to Tom*):   Your brother does.

FATHER: Why do you think I pick on you needlessly, Tom?

TOM: Needlessly?

FATHER: Yes. I pick on you for nothing?

(I lean over to the mother again and say, "That was very good. That's exactly what you need to do. Because otherwise he's going to be a mess (pointing to Mike)—he's going to be very confused.")

TOM: Sometimes.

FATHER: Like?

TOM: When you're mad at Mike, you might take it out on me, Vanessa, or Cindy, or Mom.

FATHER: When I'm mad at Mike, aren't you guys all doing something wrong when I holler?

TOM: No. Even if we aren't doing anything. When you get mad at Mike, you always take it out on us, too.

FATHER: Okay. I know what you're referring to. If I get really caught up with what Michael did, then the slightest little thing that you guys do gets me. You're correct. I'm sorry. You're correct.

> *The father's apology is the first step toward an important goal: fostering a positive regard, a respect and liking among family members. Reaching this goal will become possible as the structure begins to change and as the mother begins to support her husband.*

I ask the mother if this dispersion of antagonism happens at home. She responds "All the time." I say to her, "This is an opportunity to have things change once and for all." I leave the room; as I do, the mother puts her face in her hands.

FATHER   But you still have not answered my question as to why
(*to Mike*):   you don't like me?

MIKE: I don't. I just don't. I don't like to be near you. Probably because you do that . . .

MOTHER: Mike, do you know why it is? Because I've let Daddy take over. I've let him take that burden. That's why you don't like Daddy. Because he's had it all, all these years—not me. You wouldn't like me either then.

> *The mother realizes that she has set up her husband.*

MIKE: I wouldn't like you either?

MOTHER: No, because I've let him have it all.

MIKE: I sort of know what you've been going through silently,
and I haven't been helping much. And I admit that. And
Dad, I haven't been helping him out. I haven't been helping anybody. But I *will* now.

Much of Mike's wish to do better in school is an effort to
get out of situations where he is always considered wrong
or irresponsible.

The therapist makes an extremely important intervention to keep the
new, albeit inchoate, pattern going. She says to the mother, who again has
put her head down, "Continue. Tell him how you feel." The therapist
realizes that the forces of the old homeostasis are telling the mother—and
the therapist—to slow down, to stop this painful sequence of change. This
kind of behavior, the emergence of this new mother-father coalition, is
uncomfortable, and resistance to it is rising. So the therapist, as an agent of
change, seeks to maintain the new pattern by allowing the family a different experience with one another right here in the room.

MOTHER: But you feel like Daddy—Daddy has been the sole disciplinarian in the family. And I have made a mistake by
grouping up with you. It's been wrong. And that's why
you don't like Daddy and you do like Mommy. I mean, it's
easy to like me—what did I ever do when you did something wrong? Nothing! You'd laugh.
MIKE: Laugh at you?
FATHER: No, Michael. Mother didn't say you laugh at her.
MOTHER: You never took me seriously because I've always let
Daddy do the hard work. I've always let Daddy be the
heavy. It was very easy for me to do that. And now, when
I see the way you guys talk, and the way you say you
feel—there's no real basis for it. It's killing me right now.
It's really—it's causing me pain. Because I can't stand it. I
can't stand it anymore.

Of course, the mother's defense of her husband here is an incomplete
story. It was not *only* because she joined in a coalition against him and left
him with the main burden that the father is an aggressive trespasser and
disrespectful to his children. It was also because of the father's own irre-
sponsibility. He cannot see this because she has always taken over to cover
up for him, as she has done now. In this complex system, by not allowing

him to work out his differences with the kids directly, the mother has crippled her husband in the act of defending him. To the extent that no one has ever attacked this man for being a trespasser who picks on the kids, he does not know he must change.

The therapist must now begin to work with Mike's relationship with his father in order to enhance his feelings of self-worth. A powerful way to do this is through negotiation. But negotiation only can work if it is done from mutual respect. Can the boy negotiate not from a position of being one down and degraded, but from a position of respect? Similarly, it is clear that the father also needs to be respected to be able to live in this family.

THERAPIST:	Tell them why it hurts you.
MOTHER:	Because I know he's been trying. George has tried. He loves those children. Maybe more—as much as I. I know he does. I've seen him in pain because he's wanted to do the right thing.
MIKE:	I've never seen my father hurt in any way, except one time, and that was . . .
MOTHER:	I know—I'm telling you, I know. I have. I have seen it.
MIKE:	I've never seen it.
MOTHER:	I have.
THERAPIST:	Tell him when you've seen it.

The new pattern of mother supporting father rather than son might have become short-lived without the therapist's support to maintain its development.

MOTHER:	I've seen your father hurt every time you've done something wrong. I've seen him hurt every time that—that—when he's tried talking, and he's walked away in frustration.
MIKE:	I have never seen him.
MOTHER:	I have.

Note in the next sequence how the therapist discourages the father from entering. The change being sought is a transformation of roles: the mother taking some responsibility for discipline and in turn allowing the father to become more nurturing.

FATHER: Mike, how many times have we talked? How many times have I said to you, and to everyone else, whenever you want to discuss something, I'm here, no matter how bad it is?

THERAPIST: George, please. I would like Patty to continue telling him about this. Because they have heard this from you many times before, but not from Patty.

MOTHER: Everything Daddy has done—even though you may not think so—he has done because he loves you. He loves you.

MIKE: No. I think he's right about the studying. I'm glad—I really think I do more because of it.

MOTHER: But everything. He's done it because he cares so much. If he didn't care, he wouldn't do it. He would say, "The hell with them, I don't care. The hell with all of them." Do you think it's easy? It's not easy to do what he does. It takes a lot out of you.

MIKE: Then I won't give him any—I will try not to give him . . .

MOTHER (*crying*):   And you don't know what you do to him when you do that. You know that you take more out of him, I think, because he's the one that's put so much in—and I've stepped back and I watched it.

The stress on Mike to reform, to "show me something," amounts to wrathful projections of the father's own troubles in reforming his drinking.

MIKE: I agree with how he feels. My word's no good until I start showing something.

MOTHER: Look at what you've been doing. You've been causing so much pain in the family.

MIKE: And I will try not to.

MOTHER: Not just your father. Not just between us [the parents]— all of us. We felt it. When you ran away, your brothers and sister felt it. Our whole world was turned upside down because of you. You affected every one of us. Most of all your father. He was so upset that I didn't know what to do with him.

MIKE: But all I heard is that he hollered.

MOTHER: He didn't holler—he was scared! Because he cares so much he wants the best for you. He wants the best. I've seen him at Christmas. He's worse than me with you kids. When he saw those coats up there, he made me buy them, because he wanted his sons to have coats because you'd been complaining. And ᵗe went overboard on buying you guys clothes. It wasn't me. I was hollering at him for it. What he did was for you kids. The way he has taken his last couple of dollars to buy you kids shoes and stuff— and I hollered. But he said you were going to get shoes. And you kids were going to get haircuts before he did. He wouldn't get his hair cut because you guys needed a haircut.

At this point the father, struggling to control his emotions, gets up and kisses his wife, saying, "It's all right." The experience is obviously new for him and he is grateful that his wife had seen a side of him that he didn't know she so clearly understood. The therapist directs the father to sit down again when it appears that he is thinking of leaving the room. Spurred by his mother's revelation, Mike now goes out of his way to tell his father, "All I could see was your anger, and not your pain."

The following sequence demonstrates the emerging humanization of the father in the eyes of the family. That Mike and the other children were complaining that they saw only the dark side of their father suggests that they believed there was more and that they wanted more.

MIKE: Listen, Dad, every time something happens, or I do something wrong, you never say you are worried or hurt. You would get angry, or you wouldn't get angry. You just never showed that you were hurt or anything. You told me that it's hurting Mommy really bad. You said that it's hurting me, but it's hurting Mommy a lot more. That's what you would say to me, and that would be all with that.

FATHER: Sure you're hurting your mother. Look at her now, she's crying. The night that you wanted to leave home, she was crying. It hurts me also. Don't misunderstand. It hurts me also.

MIKE: It doesn't seem to hurt you.

FATHER: But when you're acting like that—do you leave me room to be human? How do you know what's inside of me?

MIKE: I don't. It doesn't seem like that on the outside. It doesn't.

FATHER: Then why don't you ask me?

MIKE: Why don't I ask you? How can I ask you?

FATHER: A couple of weeks ago I went up to your room after we had an argument. What did I do? I put my arms around you, and I hugged you, and I said, "Mike, I love you. And if I don't do enough of this, let me know. Is this what you need?" And you said, "Yes," did you not?

(The father gets up, crying. He kisses his wife and moves out of the circle to sit near the door.)

THERAPIST: I think that what happened just now is an indicator of what probably happens at home. You see that Patty is doing a terrific job, but you say, "This is getting too emotional for me and I'd rather step out." And you step out until you can cool off and you can come back in with your rational, cool air—or angry. But you are much more able to show your rational understanding than your emotions. And when you get too emotional, you step out until things cool off.

FATHER: Okay, I see what you are saying.

THERAPIST: So the image the children have of you is either angry or disengaged—you don't care. It's not that you don't care. It's that you care so much. And you feel so tender and so soft that you have to move out. Because you feel that if you show them how tender and soft you are, and caring, then they'll step all over you.

The mother, having proven herself available to her husband and supporting him in dealing with the youngsters, is now also able to demand strongly that the pattern between her and her husband change. In the following sequence from the next session the parents discuss problematic issues between them—disappointments, drinking, their availability to each other. The therapist deals with their renewal of their contract with each other as spouses.

MOTHER: I am afraid of that pattern starting again. It's destructive to both of us and to the family, and I am afraid of it.

FATHER: Don't you think that the fear and the moodiness that you're having is affecting the family right now?

MOTHER: Yes. It is. Yes, it is.

THERAPIST: Could you describe that pattern to me?

MOTHER: The drinking, the anger, hostility. I am afraid of the pattern starting up. And it is draining, and it's not good for both of us. Also because the next step is George is sorry. And he does come and say, "I'm wrong."

FATHER: It's not good enough.

The mother has seen through her husband's talk and now demands more of him. She is aiming for a new boundary.

MOTHER: It's not that it's not good enough. It's that I've heard it before. I've heard the awareness thing before and I've heard—I know I should be more aware—and it's just the same thing over and over again.

The therapist acts to reinforce this change in the mother.

THERAPIST: Let me tell you what I'm hearing. What I'm hearing is that you're both complaining to each other that you're not available enough to each other. We've had a lot of experience with families that have this kind of problem, and in my experience, always when one of the two members of the couple needs to go out to have fun in some way, it's because that person is not satisfied within their relationship. This is what you're both telling each other. And this is what you're both handling in different ways. George goes out to drink. You're busy with your own work. And you work a lot and then you come home and you're not available to him to the extent that he would like you to be. He complains about you not being available to the children, and not disciplining, and so forth. Which I'm sure is true. But basically what I hear is that neither of you is as available to the other as you would like.

Making these parents more available to each other meant having them focus on working together on the process of change. Following the principle of dealing with the broader context, the therapeutic team has told the family that therapy would be best conducted after they had temporarily stopped working with their respective therapists. In the following excerpt the therapist first learns that this had not yet occurred.

MOTHER: I am told to start becoming really autonomous and start finding some strength, start becoming completely, totally independent.

FATHER: But the fact that you're autonomous doesn't mean that you have to be a loner. The fact that you're autonomous means that you can handle situations. Do I have to be there every time something happens?

THERAPIST (*to the father*): You've got a point there.

MOTHER: Are you?

FATHER: When am I not?

MOTHER: George, you are not there all the time to handle situations.

FATHER: Then I get it when I come home.

MOTHER: I was told once and by several people what is wrong emotionally.

FATHER: Where?

MOTHER: In therapy. I have to start building trust. You know, ask your husband, be comfortable with him.

THERAPIST: Patty, I have one request to make of you. When you talk to George, talk about what you think and what you feel. Because if you bring in your therapist, it's like putting a third person into it.

MOTHER: Yes, I know.

From behind the mirror I call the therapist suggesting that she work with the complementary behaviors of both parents' alienating obsessions: father's drinking and mother's studies. If they could get closer as a couple then the driven quality of these activities might diminish.

THERAPIST: What I am seeing is that you are both feeling very lonely. You are both trying very hard and you don't know in what direction to pull. I would like you to try to work out now, here, something very concrete by which you both can be more available to each other.

MOTHER: Be more available to each other?

THERAPIST: You both want to make a go out of this.

MOTHER: Come home and take me out with you. I'll sit with you, have a drink with you.

FATHER: I would be willing to do that.

After this session at the suggestion of the therapist the couple went away alone on a vacation for a week. It was the first time in fourteen years that they had done this. As the husband and wife's struggle for availability to each other continued, the father, on his own, became more available to the youngsters in new areas. Near the end of therapy, about four months after the initial session, the atmosphere between children and father had changed.

THERAPIST: Are you more satisfied, more comfortable with Vanessa now?

FATHER: Oh, yeah. I'm fine with her. We had our little talk and she claims that she didn't want to talk to me because I didn't like what she would have to say. And I said to her, "Fine, well, this is your opportunity to express yourself." She said, "All right." And she sat me down and said, "I'm gonna tell you what I think." And she did. And I told her what I thought. And I think what I said made sense because she said to me, "Why are you always right?" Did I say to you that it was wrong for you to argue with me and express yourself? Did I?

VANESSA: No.

FATHER: All right, then. I listened to what you had to say, and you listened to what I had to say, and I am hoping that we resolved it. Later on when you went crying to your teacher, what did she say? "Your dad is right" (*he laughs*).

VANESSA: You're always right, Dad. I don't know how you do it (*they all laugh*).

As the father moved in the direction of availability and nurturance of the youngsters, the mother moved increasingly into unaccustomed areas of discipline and control.

MIKE: You don't think I'm being consistent in my math. There is nothing I can do about that.

MOTHER: Yes, there is. There is something you can do, but you don't want to hear any suggestions anyone can give you.

MIKE: Why should I accept suggestions? You don't think I'm doing well, that is your opinion.

MOTHER: You told me yourself you're flunking algebra.

MIKE: What I meant was, you don't think that I'm really trying, that's what you said. (*He begins to cry.*)

> *He cries because his parents do not accept his limitations*
> *and keep humiliating him.*

MOTHER: Why are you crying?

As the mother began to assert greater control, she took some of the burden of being the "bad guy" disciplinarian off her husband. The parents could control Mike when necessary, but could they also allow him a voice? The therapeutic goal was not just the establishment of an executive hierarchy that could effectively enforce rules. The goal was also for an executive authority that could negotiate with the emerging adolescents, so that the children could feel respected and free.

In the following segment from the termination session the mother describes new pathways used by the children. They used to be wedded to her; now they go to their father. These changes manifest the family structure's increasing flexibility.

THERAPIST: What are the things that you feel have been accomplished?

MIKE: Nothing. (*Everyone laughs.*)

MIKE: It's made Mom—you know—she's not going off hollering. You know, all hollering at somebody. If she's not home, my dad's there. But if he's hollering, she just goes back.

FATHER: I don't understand that one.

MIKE: It's like—when she's home you let her handle it.

FATHER: What's wrong with that?

MIKE: I didn't say there was anything wrong with it.

THERAPIST: That's changed. How do you find that things have changed, Patty?

MOTHER: With me, or with the children?

THERAPIST: With the family in general.

MOTHER: I think that they are all working harder with their homework. They are becoming more conscientious. I think that they're all looking at me twice now. In fact, one of the things I've noticed is that they don't run to me all the time. I'm still learning to block out the fighting between the kids somewhat. I'm still working on that. But they don't come to me—if their father does something. It was constant. But they don't do that any more. That has stopped completely.

THERAPIST: Did they go to you?

MOTHER: Yes. Now they won't come to me. And if they have, then it's been, "What does your father say?" That's changed.

THERAPIST: So you feel that you're both pulling together?

MOTHER: Yes. The way we've been doing things—I love it. It's taken pressure off me in one way and it's taken pressure off him in another way. There's not that tension all the time—you know. That's gone. I don't feel like there's such a burden. That's changed.

THERAPIST (*to the father*): Do you notice how much more relaxed Patty looks? The expression on her face?

FATHER: That's because she had to be out for my birthday last night.

Notice in the next sequence how the therapist enhances Mike's position in the family and normalizes his behavior as part of a developmental process that they are all engaged in.

MIKE: But how come it always has to be me and not them?

THERAPIST: You know why—because you are the eldest. And you are the one who's moving apart now. You are more on your own. Your brothers and your sister are younger than you are. And it's only logical at your age that you should think differently and react differently, have different interests. And that's part of growing up.

The therapist is emphasizing the need to respect the differences among the children. The older ones have more rights and more obligations than the younger ones. This is part of the overall goal of helping the family members to like and value one another. And with that respect and liking, the family can work toward the ultimate mission in the raising of adolescents: separation without devaluation.

FATHER: Well, not only that. There is one thing that Patty and I picked up. If he's behaving himself, and if he's being himself, so to speak—I mean I realize we were all crazy at one time, we were all teenagers. They all look—they all take the example. This one [Tommy], the older he is getting, is becoming more and more protective of this one [Mike].

MIKE: Good, I protect him, too.

FATHER: I know that—that's nice. I'm not saying there's anything wrong with that.

MIKE: So, it's no longer you and mother against each of us. It's all of us against you. If you want to put it that way.

Note that Mike has given a reading of the competing coalitions in the family.

FATHER: Oh, I love it. I love it.

MIKE: If you want to put it in terms of that . . .

MOTHER: It's lovely.

MIKE: Everybody's telling everybody they're against us, so . . .

THERAPIST: That's the way it should be. You guys have to pull together because you're siblings. And your parents have to pull together as parents.

FATHER: You know you're doing well. The only thing I said to you was that anything I discussed with you has been something that has been bad—hasn't it.

MIKE: Could we make some kind of thing here—my studying and my work and everything for school should be left to me.

FATHER: Great. Then, also right now, let's agree on something more.

MOTHER: What?

FATHER: Bedtime at a certain hour. Because, I'll be damned if you're going to stay up till 11:00 or 12:00 on a school night.

The initial presentation of this family was of a family in disarray. The therapy was aimed at the establishment of executive control and a restored interaction between the father and his children. In addition, the therapy attempted to create a parental subsystem by issuing a clear message to the parents that they needed to be in charge. In the final sequence just presented, however, we see a warning of the problems to come. Just as Mike succeeds in wresting control of his own schoolwork, his father brings up an entirely new issue: bedtime. In retrospect, the therapeutic team should not have ignored this last request. The father was backing off in one area but intrusively digging into another. The system was lapsing back to a previous structure, and the therapy should not have ended at that point. This is precisely the kind of boundary violation that, two years later, would lead the therapist to work for a radical weaning of the parents, as we will see later in this chapter.

THE FOLLOW-UP

Initially this family system seemed to be one in which the causal problem was an overintrusive father. But it became apparent in therapy that the difficulties were more complex. The mother's coalition with her children was a means to establish a defensive alliance against her abusive husband. However, that very coalition also pushed the father into his role as an unloved enforcer of rules. After a great deal of work this dysfunctional system was effectively changed. There was a structural shift: the father learned to pull out of his role of angry disciplinarian and taskmaster and was restored to the family center. He began to be more mindful of the children in a different way, relieving his wife of some of the caretaking. This was not a comfortable change for him and he did it with hesitancy and questionable authority, but he did it. That transformation was essential in order to put a stop to the family's violence.

During the follow-up we found new problems emerging. The family accepted that the structural transformation was an honest one, but also found it difficult to uphold. Unaccustomed to her new role, the mother had become a "furious witch" in trying to contain the children. And the father was now perceived as a "hollow wall"; he made noises and gestures of controlling his children, but no one in the family really respected him.

The new structure was an oddly layered one. The pattern of violence had been suppressed and the youngsters were not as intimidated. But there was still edginess and touchiness. The children sensed that the one in authority had no right to be in control. Clearly, this issue of rightful authority and the observance of mutual responsibilities and boundaries remained a constant, fundamental problem within this family.

The next sequence is from the first follow-up session, held two months after the therapy had ended. The family continues to struggle with their changes. Strain has developed.

> *Notice how the mother expresses her own fears about the changes in her husband, which she feels uncertain about.*

MOTHER: George and I are fighting to work out our problems. It's a lot of effort going into it, it really is. George has enrolled in a technical college. He's starting school in January and I'm really proud of him. And his drinking—it has gone down to almost rare—he does not drink like he used to. I still have fears—a tremendous fear. But I see that he's not going to get angry and hostile, and destroy the family. Now when I see consistently that it isn't happening, it's almost like I could make it happen because of my fear. And I'm trying to know that when he goes out, he's going to be okay when he comes home. He's not going to be drunk. He won't admit it.

FATHER: What won't I admit to?

MOTHER: He's been really trying. But it's been hard for him after all the time that's passed to understand that the fear can't leave just like that. It's very strong. We're working on it.

FATHER: Honey, we had a conversation about that once before. What did I say to you? I am not really putting a hell of a lot of effort into this. I'm not.

MOTHER: You did say that to me.

FATHER: Okay, I'm not.

MOTHER: That you're being nice because it's coming natural.

FATHER: Because it's just me. And I even asked you to stop and think about it. If you recall this past winter, you're right. I was a pain in the ass, literally. But that was last winter.

MOTHER: And when you came home that day and I was all upset. When something like that happens, I get like—you know the fear. And you are prepared for it and you're on the defensive when you come home.

FATHER: Not really, I haven't been.

MOTHER: It's because you're losing patience with me.

FATHER: I think it's a little ridiculous at times.

MOTHER: And it does put me into depression from time to time. Sometimes it takes me a couple of days to get out of it. It's just a fear of what can happen and what may happen. Really, I'm trying not to do that. I'm trying to take one day at a time.

The central transformation in this family was the father's foregoing his harsh disciplinarian stance and becoming friendlier and more nurturing to his children. This had two results: the children were able to establish their own turf in the family, and the mother took over the unaccustomed function of being in charge. Both changes were possible because the parents were in the process of resolving their difficulties as husband and wife and were no longer involving their children to diffuse the conflict. Mike's problems became manageable after he was freed from the coalition, and he was able to work on his own developmental issues. The couple was now struggling with coordinating individual growth as they both went to school while maintaining child-rearing responsibilities.

The family was seen for another follow-up seven months later. The following sequence is from that session.

THERAPIST: And Mike?

MOTHER: I wish he had come here tonight so you could have seen him. You won't believe the change.

FATHER: The kid on the tape is not the Mike now.

MOTHER: It is not. Just a total complete turnabout. It was rough going, don't get me wrong. We have our arguments and everything, but it's nothing like before. His marks have improved. His attitude—he's much more free, he's much more open, he's much more expressive. When George and Mike talk there's no tension. It's comfortable. They communicate. There's no heavy, hard anger. It's just so different.

THERAPIST: That was happening toward the end already.

FATHER: Yes. But he doesn't walk out—if I start to push. He'll say—okay, okay, Dad, let's talk about it.

MOTHER: His relationship with his father has changed to a point where sometimes I feel like I'm left out. I don't voice it—I'm okay. But, he wants his Dad. And I really love that. My son Thomas says he wants to talk to Dad. It's such a difference. But you've changed, George. You've changed. You're not as authoritarian, angry, tyrant. You're not like that. You're much more sensitive.

FATHER: I don't have to be a tyrant, I hear about how bad you are.

MOTHER: So, that makes you calm down.

FATHER: That makes me calm down. I feel why the hell should I do it (*he laughs*).

THERAPIST: That's something you have to pay attention to.

MOTHER: I know that.

THERAPIST: Because you're both growing, but you have to be growing in a way that you're both interlocked.

MOTHER: Exactly.

FATHER: I compromise. It's like when I came back from my side
           job. Report cards were being given out and parents had to
           pick up the report cards. What did I say to you? "I'm
           going."

MOTHER: Yes, you did.

FATHER: I went with you.

MOTHER: Oh, yes, you did.

FATHER: I wasn't up to it.

MOTHER: We don't need the extra money. We could make it without
           it. We've done it before. It would be tight. But it's tight
           with him working the side job. But he'd be home more.
           His mind is one-track right now. All he's thinking is the
           money. And he's right in one way, and I'm right in my
           way.

FATHER: I never said you were wrong. I agree with you. It would be
           nice if I didn't have to work weekends. What makes you
           think I want to?

MOTHER: Sometimes I don't think you realize how important it is for
           us to be together.

This is a case that argues vividly for a therapy that goes beyond the
crisis induction and resolution stage, a therapy that monitors the changes
in such a way that they do not ossify, creating further pathology in a
different form somewhere down the line. The outstanding characteristic of
this family was a tendency to make rigid whatever gains they attained. As
a result, after one crisis was past, another was often created.

The next phase of the therapy began two years after the last session,
when the family called asking for additional help. They were having difficulties with the children, and I agreed to see them the following week.
Assembled in the room: mother, father, and the kids. Mike was now
seventeen, Tom sixteen, Vanessa thirteen, and Cindy twelve. I was now
the primary therapist since the supervisee had moved.

During this session the task of the therapist was to facilitate the disengagement of the parents from the children. This disengagement depends
on getting the parents to recognize the legitimacy of focusing on their own
goals instead of totally submerging themselves in their responsibility for
their children's schooling. Once this recognition is accomplished, the therapy begins to move much further in maintaining the necessary changes in
the family's structure.

MOTHER: We've been having a lot of difficulty since we've been here. This has been going on. It seems like when George and I gang up on them to study, they'll study. But if we're not on their backs, as soon as they feel they can relax, they do.

DR. FISHMAN: All right, I hear you now, but let's go back.

As I began the session, I questioned whether this was in fact an identical dysfunctional system. Were mother and father completely split? Had they relapsed into being a very unhappy family, or was this instead just a single area of isolated conflict? It soon became clear that the original therapy should have ended with absolutely clear boundaries established for the issue of the children's schooling, because the parents themselves were both struggling to complete their own educations and were thus extremely focused on school.

FATHER: The kids for some reason or other feel that Mom and Dad are supposed to wipe their little tails continuously. This is what Patty meant when she said that we were still having similar problems. This is the only part that basically has remained.

DR. FISHMAN: What are the other things?

FATHER: This is the first time also that all four of them have brought home failures. This is the main reason, plus the fact that Mike is up to his old tricks of cutting school, cutting classes.

MOTHER: This is the third year. We found out again last week that he has been cutting.

FATHER: Other than that . . .

MOTHER: There's not much of any problems. It's been okay, nothing like before, it's just schoolwork.

DR. FISHMAN: When you say nothing like before, what has stopped?

MOTHER: Well, I have taken a more assertive role; I am not totally assertive, George does have to help, but I have become more assertive. Now I find myself hollering a lot and when I see him get upset I try to come in. Before I would let him do it all.

DR. FISHMAN: What else has changed?

FATHER: Patty and I usually discuss what we are going to do with the kids, what our plans should be with them. But it seems that every time we bend over backward, both of us, we get it socked to us.

DR. FISHMAN: What does "socked to you" mean?

MOTHER: Well, their grades, they tell us we are not fair, and . . .

FATHER: Everybody else is at fault but them.

MOTHER: Right. Oh, when I get angry, even still to this day they can't handle it. I'm mean and they'll go to their father and say, "Calm Mommy down, she is mad again. She's angry all the time."

DR. FISHMAN: What do you do?

FATHER: I usually ask them what her reason for being angry is. This way I hear their side of the story. And nine out of ten times, if she is upset the kids and I will speak. And normally, I can see. Vanessa was the most recent one when Mom was upset because she thought she was unfair and we sat and spoke and she saw where Mom was coming from and that she was being fair. This is what usually happens.

DR. FISHMAN: So you feel supported by your husband?

MOTHER: Oh, he does support me. And I don't support him, I must say, as much as he does me. There are still times I have difficulty, when I see and accept it.

FATHER: It's not as often as it used to be.

MOTHER: I don't give 100 percent, I say like 80 percent of the time.

DR. FISHMAN: Could you agree 80 percent?

FATHER: Like I said, it's not like it used to be before.

MOTHER: When it was like 5 percent of the time.

FATHER: But what really brought us is that I have been noticing Mike's behavior and I caught a few things that were strange to me, as a father.

The feeling in the room is much different from when they first came to therapy. It was much lighter. By now all feelings about the father as a possible "ax murderer" have vanished; that kind of poisonous atmosphere is not present. Nonetheless, the family is not completely happy. The parents are struggling very hard to get their children to do better in school, as they themselves are trying to do. But they see only poor grades, absenteeism, and lack of effort.

The main issue for the present therapy is developmental estrangement. The more the parents pressured their children around school, the more the children rebelled and did poorly, and the more confused they were about for whom and what they were in school. We proceed by looking at what in the parents' experience causes them to focus on school so much.

DR. FISHMAN *(to the mother)*:	Where are you now, still in nursing school?
MOTHER:	I'm still in nursing school.
DR. FISHMAN:	How is that going?
MOTHER:	I have eighteen months to go, very stressful. Other than that it is going fine.

(At this point the father has a spell of heavy coughing.)

DR. FISHMAN:	How are you, George?
FATHER:	I'm still working as a clerk and going to school at night.
DR. FISHMAN:	What are you studying?
FATHER:	Computers. Hopefully, if they ever cut me a break and let me spend the time with it I need.
DR. FISHMAN:	Who are "they"?
FATHER:	My kids.

The parents' reaction suggests stress in the family system. When the mother said school was "very stressful," the father coughed vigorously. The father, when asked about his own career, said he would be doing fine in his schoolwork if the kids would let him. Clearly, the parents were struggling in school as they desperately tried to recapture lost time. The father's frustration regarding his difficulty in focusing on school will become important information for the therapist later in the session, when it is necessary to create a boundary between the parents and their children's schooling.

It is also interesting to note that at this point there is reportedly no more violence in the family. In a sense, however, there is some of the same intrusiveness and the same sense of helplessness on both sides. The overfocusing on school created a suppressed rage, although to a lesser extent than before. Clearly, an intervention is necessary to increase a sense of control around this issue for both parents and children.

DR. FISHMAN:	You guys are working pretty hard.
MOTHER:	They keep you working.
DR. FISHMAN:	Why are you working so hard?

I begin an attempt to get these parents to see that their constant intrusiveness had not been successful.

MOTHER: We are trying to keep them on the right road, we want them to do well for life, for the future. It counts now.

DR. FISHMAN: Has it been successful?

MOTHER   Not with her it hasn't.
(indicating
Vanessa):

DR. FISHMAN: Yes, but she is so young.

MOTHER: She's thirteen. No, I know what you mean. It hasn't worked, no.

DR. FISHMAN: It sounds like you've been working very hard.

FATHER: And getting nowhere.

DR. FISHMAN: Something that you said really struck home. You said that your school plans are being curtailed by all the work that you are doing for these kids.

FATHER: Yes. Because I have to be home, I have to be around, I have to check on homework.

DR. FISHMAN: You know something? Maybe you don't.

As the session proceeds I continue to explore the parents' feelings about whether what they are doing is successful and whether it may be impeding their own careers.

During the original course of therapy this family was characterized by the youngsters' readiness to jump into angry or violent behavior. To further probe the system I challenge Mike, who is still the most problematic of these four adolescents, by asking a series of challenging, almost sarcastic, questions, to test the extent to which he might still be ready to engage in violent expression.

DR. FISHMAN: So he won't go to a school for the academically talented. Maybe he will decide to live with another family in another school district.

MOTHER: That is up to him.

DR. FISHMAN: This young man is a part-time student there at high school. (To Mike:) Next year you will probably be at public school.

MIKE: I wish you wouldn't say anything. I'm asking—like I'm not—you know . . . (He is upset.)

DR. FISHMAN: Well, then, you tell me the truth.

As I exacerbate the system, the boy attacks.

MIKE:	What do you mean? What do you want me to say? I wish you would stop exaggerating things—you've done it, like, twice already.
DR. FISHMAN:	What am I exaggerating?
MIKE (*to Dr. Fishman*):	You're banging around the "part-time" student—real smart remarks. Like—I don't deserve—and I don't even know you. (*To his father:*) I'm sorry I had to say it here. This is open and I had to tell him.

The father attempts to deflect the attack and come to the rescue. But Mike won't allow it. He then apologizes to his father for getting out of hand.

The extent to which Michael felt offended by the intruding adults is apparent. My sarcasm and provocative challenge brought out the fact that this is a young man with a very large chip on his shoulder and that his father cannot effectively apply brakes to his son's behavior. From this testing of the patterns of violence it is apparent that the therapy must aim for a radical weaning of the parents from the children.

DR. FISHMAN:	Between us, so you are going to school every day?
MIKE:	Yes.
DR. FISHMAN:	What I mean by part time is that I thought you were only going to school four days a week rather than five. Because that is kind of like a part-time employee. Forgive me if I am wrong; I would not want to misrepresent it, because you are right, I don't know you.
MIKE:	But it's like this. It was in February and I took off on Fridays. My marks—if my dad would have spoken to the teachers at that particular time—when he called, I wished he would have, because they would have told him last week.
DR. FISHMAN:	I was only saying that you are a part-time student, it is what I heard, that you were only going four days a week. To me that is part-time. Is that a misrepresentation?
MIKE:	From what?
DR. FISHMAN:	From whatever point. Was that a misrepresentation?
MIKE:	It depends on what—I suppose he could be right.

Mike's facial expressions and gestures show a young man about to blow up. He is angry.

DR. FISHMAN: I didn't want to be disrespectful.

> *I use the opportunity to say what this youngster has long needed to hear from his parents: "I didn't want to be disrespectful."*

Having violated boundaries through sarcasm, I realized that I had better make repairs. But the situation was not without advantage. By first offending the boy and then making repairs, I could establish a model for the father, who thought himself effective only when vociferous in making his displeasure known. So I use the opportunity to show that an adult can make an error and then retract and repair it.

MIKE: I know I asked you . . .
DR. FISHMAN: Good. I appreciate it.
MIKE: Now if he would have gone and talked to my teachers, it was like I . . .
DR. FISHMAN: You don't have to talk to me about it.
MIKE: No. (*To his father:*) No, but if you had gone and talked to my teachers—I wished you would have because you would have heard what they have to say.
DR. FISHMAN: You know, I want to apologize to you. I was kind of probing you, hassling you and saying that I think you were wrong in going only four days a week, but you know something? I was wrong in saying that. You know why?

> *I go out of my way to highlight this because it is a new message for these parents. In addition, I am honestly responding to the young man's fury. I really was sorry.*

MIKE: Why?
DR. FISHMAN: Because it is up to you. If you want to go four days a week, it is up to you. I apologize. It is up to you.

> *This is a long-awaited response that the young man had been trying to extract from his father. I thus create an option, a behavior alien but necessary to this system, and I do so quite pointedly in front of the father, who needs to learn it.*

What is demonstrated here is the salve that is needed but rarely supplied in systems that are prone to violence: offering apologies, soothing hurt feelings, requesting forgiveness. For this essential behavior to begin, the therapist has to model it.

In the last sequence the young man was invited to reflect on why I was wrong. When he was ready, and only when he was ready—when he asked "why?"—then I responded: "Because it is up to you." This is a family that does not prize autonomy. Therefore, the therapist must prize it in the hope that the parents will learn to appreciate and respect the children's independence.

In working toward weaning the parents from their children I have established a necessary sense of apology and respect and focus the therapy on the reorganization of values in the system and the restoring of choice, specifically on Mike's having a choice concerning his performance in school. It is clear that if his parents continued to steal his choice and press the issue, violence might emerge. So I work to stay on track, tenaciously reiterating the necessity of choice.

DR. FISHMAN *(to the parents)*:	The more you've done, the less they've done.
MOTHER:	That's true. That is true.
DR. FISHMAN:	I mean, they are fine kids. They may just not do very well in school, but that is all right
MOTHER:	But can you allow that, how can you?
DR. FISHMAN:	Well, talk to your husband about the alternatives.
FATHER:	This is the one thing that . . .
MIKE:	In our house it's always school this and school that. It is constantly like that. I'm not putting it down, but, they just want us to have a better life than they did and . . .
DR. FISHMAN:	But you know something? There is no reason. How old are you now?
FATHER:	Thirty-six.
DR. FISHMAN:	There is no reason why at thirty-five they can't go back to school too. Why should they be any different from you? At what age did you drop out of school?
FATHER:	I made first semester of college and then dropped out.
DR. FISHMAN:	So maybe they'll do that. You are a young man at thirty-five.
FATHER:	They can do that at thirty-five.
DR. FISHMAN:	I'm suggesting that there is nothing you can do.

*The aim here is to help the parents let go and break the
entrapment. In this kind of therapy it is extremely important to understand that the therapist is not playing games.
I am sincere when I suggest that there is nothing they can
do. This is not a ploy. It is an attempt to convey a real
truth.*

FATHER: I realize what you are saying, but at the same time I made
my point on numerous occasions. It is not that we are
asking for that much.

MOTHER: There is nothing we can do. You don't feel there's anything we can do, doctor.

DR. FISHMAN: What you can do is to work harder on your own work so
that your careers are functioning. The more you have
done, the fewer results you have gotten. (*To the children:*)
The more your parents have done, the worse you are
getting. Would you agree? The more your parents have
tried to help you in school?

MIKE: Yeah.

DR. FISHMAN: The more they do, the less they get what they want. (*To
the parents:*) They can be happy. At thirty-five they can go
back to school.

FATHER: There is nothing out there.

DR. FISHMAN: That's only twenty years, right? You guys will be happy
and you'll be professional people and you'll be having a
good time.

FATHER: That reminds me of a conversation you [Mike] had with
me a few months ago. Where he would be content dropping out of school, working at a deli.

MIKE: I didn't say I would be content.

FATHER: If you had stayed in school I would have given you the
money you wanted; you could have done a lot more.

*The Father again becomes the harping, nagging father
and immediately gets Mike into a defensive posture. This
is the persistent quality of the dysfunctional system: all
this work, and still the father shows up with another
demand.*

MIKE: I talked about it, I did. I mentioned it, I did mention it.

DR. FISHMAN: That's fine. Sure, a lot of people work in delis. Maybe you
can work in the grocery store.

MIKE:	It sounds like you're being sarcastic again.
DR. FISHMAN:	Not at all. I'm not.
MOTHER:	He can't do it.
MIKE:	People do, they work anywhere.
DR. FISHMAN:	Of course.
MOTHER:	That's their prerogative.
DR. FISHMAN:	Your parents are very concerned about their own careers. That doesn't mean that you guys have to be.
VANESSA:	Doctor, I'm scared for him [Mike], I'm scared to death. I'm scared for him.

Notice the pattern within the family. As I wean the father, Vanessa enters and immediately fills the vacuum. This means that the weaning process has begun.

DR. FISHMAN:	You don't have to be his father.

The parents are being removed, and the test that it is effective is that the sibling steps in. Now, of course, it is necessary to get the sibling out.

This sibling reaction is typical of the breakup of intrusive systems. The moment the therapist has some effectiveness in weaning parents from children, somebody else in the system, often the sibling next in line, steps in to intrude, worry, or exercise control. There seems to be a family rule that someone is always ready to step onto another's turf, to make pronouncements about what should or should not be done. It is the exercise of this extraordinary family rule that can create an atmosphere of suffocation that leads to violence. The following sequence illustrates just such a pattern.

DR. FISHMAN:	Talk to him about it.
VANESSA (*to Mike*):	Tell me the truth—what do you want to be when you grow up? Tell the truth. Do you want to be something stupid or something smart? Or a little guy selling things in a booth?
MIKE:	I don't think you are stupid just because you don't go to school.
DR. FISHMAN:	I agree with you, of course not. You probably will have a very good job and be making lots of money, maybe they'll come to you for a loan. You have to think about that. (*To Vanessa:*) You don't have to be his mother. You are doing what your parents do. You don't have to worry about that. (*To Mike:*) They'll come to you for a loan some day.

MIKE: Or maybe you won't.

DR. FISHMAN (*to the parents*): The two of you need to let them worry about their careers. They already said that the more you do the worse results you get. You're young people, you have your whole careers ahead of you. Don't let them drag you down when really, the more you do the more you drag each other down.

MIKE: And the more angry my father gets.

MOTHER (*to Mike*): I remember I told you once, "Honey, I didn't go to school, I'm turning out pretty damn well." It was hard, damn hard, and that's when you stopped trying and relaxed, and it got to a point where there was nothing we could do, remember? That is why we called Dr. Fishman. What are we going to do this time? We didn't have any notion of what to do. We tried everything that we could possibly think of.

DR. FISHMAN: Talk about going cold turkey [in dropping their pressure on the school issue] so you won't be so tormented. Maybe show them a little respect.

As I press the parents to disengage, unconsciously I treat them like addicts. This is a family with an addictive father who in turn has created an addictive set of intruders around him.

FATHER: Up to about fifteen minutes ago I would have said no.

Note that when I have been successful at zeroing in on a significant process, it takes on a life of its own. In the next segment the father, mother, and children work at the issue strictly by themselves. There is a momentum here, and it doesn't have to be pushed along at all.

MOTHER: From now on it's their responsibility. Do you think you can do it? Let's try it. Do you know the burden that will be taken off of us? What will we do with all our spare time? You and I, what do we talk about most of the time?

FATHER: The kids.

MOTHER: Always. We rarely talk about anything else. What are we going to do about this, the report card and school. Always. We never have each other say, "Hi, how are you?"

FATHER: What happened Sunday morning?

MOTHER: We got out.

FATHER: It was the first time in years that I said, "Come on, Patty, we're going to spend the morning by ourselves away from them."

MOTHER: Do you think you can do it?

FATHER: I'm willing to try.

MOTHER: I'll help you, because there is nothing else that we can do. If somebody says to me, "Do you think you did everything you could?" I mean I sat and studied with them, I memorized the stuff. I don't know what else we can do. I just don't know. Don't you think?

FATHER: I don't know how often we ask them, if there is a problem, to come to us—and they never do.

MOTHER: Exactly. They don't. A thousand times we said, "Boys, I'm there." They know you've shown them. Have they come to you?

FATHER: No.

MOTHER: How many times have I told them, "If you're having problems outlining, come to me and I'll teach you." Have they ever come to me?

FATHER: No.

MOTHER: I go to them. You go to them. We say, "Hey, guys." And look what we find out, always the same thing. George, we'll have so much spare time, I don't know what to do with it.

CINDY: When school isn't brought up, we always have a good time, don't we?

> *This is a very important interjection. Cindy reveals that school is the loaded issue that destroys happiness in the family. Except for the issue of school—the one issue that constantly reminds them that they are failing one another —they are a very happy family. I see this remark as an extremely good prognostic sign that there is a rich sustaining fabric in this family; if we can only create a boundary around school issues, then both parents and children will be freed from an intense source of stress.*

Cindy's observation implies that there are real positives in this family. In dealing with a family system that is prone to violence, we find that the system has an undercurrent of degradation and loss of self-esteem, pride, and appreciation of who one is. What this child is really saying is this: "We do have something worthwhile somewhere, don't we?" An important part of the therapy in treating violence-prone systems is the restoration of a sense of well being and worth as a family unit. Weaning these parents is not only structurally necessary to prevent violence, it is necessary also to enable them to discover that they can like and respect one another.

An important quality of this session is that the therapy moved into the area of self-esteem. The family needs to see a positive result from its difficult attempt to break old patterns. By removing the degrading stimulus—that is, the parents' attacking the kids on the issue of school—we restore a sense of well-being. It is not, then, just a question of preserving the autonomy of the children; it is also a matter of enhancing the atmosphere for the entire family.

> FATHER: From now on there are going to be periods where your mom and I just have time for ourselves. When your friends come over you don't want us around you, do you?
>
> CINDY: No, no, it's the way you said it. The thing is, we always talk about something, when we go shopping or something like that, we always have a really good time.
>
> MOTHER: That's true.
>
> CINDY: But school is not brought up. When it is, you get very upset.
>
> FATHER: I think the problem is that Mom and I have been trying to push you guys so that you guys don't make the same mistakes we made. If you guys want to screw up now, you don't have to worry about it. No pushing of any kind in regard to school. There are going to be set chores laid down in the house that are expected to be done, period.
>
> DR. FISHMAN: That involves everybody. But schoolwork belongs to each one.
>
> MOTHER: It's their responsibility, I told them.
>
> FATHER: You flunk another one, you cry alone, I won't be there.
>
> DR. FISHMAN: You two will be out having fun.
>
> CINDY: I always come to you when I need help, but sometimes I already know it.
>
> FATHER: I've been impatient with you only when you wanted me to work out your problems, and you haven't attempted to try to do them. You expect every single answer from me. You don't sit down and try and do it on your own. That is when I get impatient with you; that is when I holler at you to get in here and try it.

CINDY:	I tried it, Dad. Mother, can I ask you a question? You guys go your own way, but I want them to help me. Okay, Mom?
FATHER:	We're there for all of you.
MOTHER:	I'll be there, but I'm not going to bat my head against the wall anymore.
DR. FISHMAN:	Do you guys have any time to go away on weekends?
MOTHER:	No, we don't go away. We don't spend, I'll tell you, any time on ourselves. We don't do anything together, we don't go anywhere.
MIKE:	You really should, because I know how hard you guys really work in school.
DR. FISHMAN *(to the father)*:	You used to drink a lot. Do you still?
VANESSA:	No.
MOTHER:	When he goes, he goes all the way. All the way. You tell him.
FATHER:	Normally I'll come home and I'll go to bed, but the reason I think everyone is laughing about it is because I came home and got in an argument with her.
MIKE:	He'll come home either really happy or really, really angry.
DR. FISHMAN:	How often is this?
CINDY:	It's practically every day.
FATHER:	Not every day.
CINDY:	I said practically every day.
MOTHER:	That is not true.
CINDY:	I know it's not true, Mom.
DR. FISHMAN:	Wait, tell your dad.
VANESSA:	Remember he came home, he brought me and my brother a cake—that was when he was really happy.
FATHER:	What happened the last time I did this, which was—what—about a month ago or a couple of weeks ago. What did I say? They got to me in the kitchen and they spoke their piece to me. Vanessa, I have to admit, put it the best, and she did it very respectfully also—and I admire her for that. She handled herself in a very mature fashion.
VANESSA:	I mean it, too, if he ever comes home that way again, that's it. I'm not going to have any more respect for him.
FATHER:	She also told me that under the conditions and in that state she has no respect for me; she was very honest. Everyone was afraid I was going to clobber them.

DR. FISHMAN: There was no clobbering.
MOTHER: No.

The family is still working on the father's recovery from alcoholism and his recovery of his children's respect. As the session continues, we proceed with the task of disengagement.

DR. FISHMAN: Are you going to be able to do it? Cold turkey?
MOTHER: Honestly, I don't know. I think I can.
DR. FISHMAN: I agree with you. I think you can, but I am wondering about your husband.
MOTHER: I am too. I really will have to—you'll have to talk to me when you feel like you are slipping.
FATHER: It hurts to see them failing.
DR. FISHMAN: I think there will be a crisis, I think one of them will come home with F's, but as long as they realize it is up to them, they will learn from their experience. Don't worry about it. Then they can go to school when they're thirty-five.
MOTHER: You feel they will bring their own grades up?
DR. FISHMAN: I think there is nothing you can do. But what you can really do is to work on your own careers. That is the only part of your family you can directly affect. Right now you can't really spend more time on their homework. They said it themselves: the less you do, the better they will do, because they'll realize that they are in it for themselves.
MOTHER: What if he fails the special high school? They don't mess around. You get a couple F's and you're out.
DR. FISHMAN: He'll take summer school.
MOTHER: They throw you out.
DR. FISHMAN: So he finds another school. Don't worry about it. If he gets kicked out of school, it will be another crisis, and he might realize what it is he needs to do for himself.

Thus I continued to encourage developmental estrangement. Once the children stopped rebelling through school and realized that school was indeed their own issue—that their parents would not rescue them—they would buckle down. In the past the school issue had been connected with pushing against their parents' authority, giving them the false illusion that they were gaining by not studying. If that false sense of gain were removed through parental distancing and the establishment of functional boundaries, the family could then get back to focusing on other, more positive issues that would help restore the mutual respect and liking that were the intended outcomes of the therapy.

Summary

When I reflect on this family I am only guardedly optimistic about how they will fare. There are so many unsettled developmental areas that are in flux. There are the adolescent and young adulthood pressures as well as pressures on the parents, who are so much in flux, both seeking new careers, and perhaps attempting to get a chance at an adolescence of their own.

However, one can also argue for optimism. This family readily seeks help in turbulent seas. I conceive of the family therapist's role as analogous to that of a family doctor who gets a family through one crisis and is available should another occur. This seems a more realistic concept than saying to the family, "Now that you have had a course of treatment, you are immune to difficulties." The systems that all of us live in are too complex and too unpredictable to offer any such smug assurances.

6

Incest: A Therapy of Boundaries

> . . . at night my father would lie with my mother. Some-
> times, I still wouldn't have fallen asleep. I'd just be lying there
> in front of her and my father would be lying down behind her
> and I would watch. At first it didn't make me unhappy. But
> once I was older I started to think, "Why doesn't my father
> care that I might still be up? I'm fairly old now, why isn't he
> being more respectful of me? Adults should be concerned
> about others. Can't they see I'm not sleeping? Why is he lying
> with her?"
>
> —!Kung Tribes-woman

IN MOST CULTURES childhood involves not only a period of sexual experimentation but also a sense of privacy about sex. Both must be respected by parents. Children may feel hurt when their parents make sexual noises in their presence; they consider it a violation of boundaries. As family therapists we must go beyond the distorted belief that lack of repression is good in all situations—a concept that has influenced much thinking on sexuality. Family therapy theory, which is attuned to the necessity for boundaries, speaks more to the issue of sexual transgression within families.

Over the last decade the extent to which children are sexually abused both within and outside of family life has become increasingly apparent, and sexual abuse is now considered a very significant problem. David

Finkelhor (1979) found that "19 percent of women and 9 percent of men report an experience of sexual abuse that appears to have had long-term harmful effects on self-image and the ability to make sexual relationships" (p. 83). Other researchers have found an even higher proportion of cases. Russell (1983) discovered that 30 percent of women reported an experience of sexual abuse before the age of eighteen and 28 percent before the age of fourteen. Such figures are alarming. We should keep in mind, however, that the term "sexual abuse" covers a wide variety of possible violations.

The focus in this chapter is incest. Freud chose to misinterpret this abuse in the sexual life of families, seeing it as a problem of repressed fantasy instead of an actual event. Why he should have done so has been the subject of much recent speculation and controversy. However, it seems clear that as a Victorian he took a position that allowed him to navigate the professional world of his times.

Today the problem of incest, though certainly more out in the open, is as difficult as ever for families to deal with. Incest often presents an extreme of suffering and illness. The issue for the therapist is the inability of the family to mobilize appropriate coalitions to defend the child. Theoretically, if, say, a father has an impulse toward incest there should be strong controls emanating not only from this man but also from the mother to prevent harm to the child. When these walls of control break down, incest is much more likely to occur. It is this rupture in family walls—that is, in the internal organization of the family—that leads to incest and its resulting pathology. As therapists we need to focus on clarifying internal boundaries and the ways in which coercion contributes to the pathology. It is the coercion, after all, that does not allow relationships to be truly symmetrical, that abuses the family hierarchy and assumes parity where none exists, and that prevents justice from reigning in the politics of the family.

General Principles

PROTECTING THE CHILD

Our first responsibility as helpers is to make sure the incestuous behavior is not repeated. Our priorities are, foremost, the protection of the child, *then* the transformation of the family system. Incest is one clinical problem where the family therapist must address the issue immediately, for it is almost always extremely destructive. But we must keep in mind that family therapy does not offer magical therapeutic cures. Therapists must realize that intervention may not necessarily put a stop to the problem. And even if the incest should cease within the current family, we cannot be sure that it will not recur in another community, when the abuser moves on and picks up another family and another child. Incest— and sexual abuse in general—presents patterns that are very difficult to change. As a result therapists must work closely with the legal authorities both to increase the force for change and to protect the child during the early stages of treatment.

In dealing with incest the family therapist treats not only the family but the larger system. Our job is to transform the system so that the incest is stopped, even if this means that the family has to be atomized and that the therapist emerges as an unfriendly consultant. Incest is the ultimate violation of boundaries, and the therapeutic work must concentrate more on repairing boundaries than on maintaining an intact family. The family therapist sees the family as a system of relationships whose purpose is to uphold the growth and health of those who compose the system. If the system of relationships fails in that job, the individual is the priority.

WINNING THE BATTLE FOR INITIATIVE

One of the key principles in treating incestuous families involves what Carl Whitaker calls the "battle for initiative" in which the therapist struggles against the family's inclination to let the therapist change them (personal communication, Feb. 1982). The battle for the therapist is to make the family *take* the initiative so that, as Whitaker says, "the family maintains total control of their life and life decisions. The family also determines what is discussed in the therapy hour and is responsible for initiating any changes in the family system" (quoted in Neill and Kniskern 1982, 213). When the problem is incest, the family must come to *own* the problem—to have the existential realization that in spite of all the helpers who are involved in their lives, the problem resides in *their family* and that the family must act to overcome it. The family must see that it is in their hands to seize the initiative and begin working toward change.

A THERAPY OF EXPERIENCE

As noted in chapter 5, one cannot assume that the violence will not recur. The same is true for incest. In spite of our best therapeutic efforts, this uncertainty will persist unless we can at least witness an actual change of behavior in the treatment room. As with violence, a therapy of experience is essential. What we look for in the therapy room are dysfunctional patterns residing within the family as well as in other elements of the system, including, if appropriate, any individual therapists. Once identified, these dysfunctional patterns are immediately challenged. If change occurs, that is an indication that the system may indeed be sufficiently flexible to move in a positive direction. If, on the other hand, the system proves intractable, as in the clinical case that follows, then we must conclude that there is a greater probability that the incest will be repeated.

In cases such as the one described in this chapter, the parents were impermeable. They had the ability to talk about changing when somebody is looking—the court, the agency, the therapist—but that did not mean they were changing. In dealing with incest it is important to consider that you may be dealing with people who are extremely clever at protecting the premises of self and are not willing to change. Thus, we need a therapy that can quickly reach those premises.

EXPOSING DARK CORNERS

In treating incestuous families some individual work must be done to help the victimized self rework the sense of trauma. I believe it is necessary for the victim to have individual sessions with someone of the same gender to work in the dark corners and to help neutralize and detoxify the memory.* It may also be necessary for individual work to be done with the other family members, especially the mother. At the heart of all pathology resulting from incest is a psychic numbness to coercion. It is important, therefore, to work with all coerced family members to undo the damage.

Often the mother has also been abused and needs to feel defended, or she feels guilty. It is also possible that the mother may be too lax about any guilt she may bear over being an accomplice to the abuse. Frequently such women have no capacity for self-assertion or for maintaining boundaries, even for simply saying "no." Like their daughters, they must be helped out of the dark. They must come to realize they have options other than coerced silence. Further, they must learn to put the right priority on their children's well-being and to defend not only themselves but their children.

It is, however, acontextual to merely dismiss the mothers as having "no capacity for self assertion." The therapist must examine the mother's contemporary context to see what relationships are giving her the sense of

---

* Clinicians are of two minds regarding the gender of the therapist for this work. Some people believe therapy should start with a therapist of the same gender because there would be more freedom to share what happened. On the other hand, it is not with persons of the same gender that the victim is likely to have difficulties. Having a therapist whose gender is the same as that of the offender could serve as a model or template for a more functional, respectful relationship.

incompetence or powerlessness. Certainly the marriage, but beyond that, for example, what about the mother's family of origin? The family needs to be included in her therapy.

BEING ALERT TO DANGER TO THE OUTSIDE CONTEXT

Incest should be viewed as a phenomenon that involves more than the nuclear family. One therapist was working with a family in which the coercive father had moved out of the state. At the end of a session with the mother, a trainee who had observed the session told the therapist that he was treating the father for the same problem in another state. The man had simply moved, established a relationship with another family, and repeated the offense.

The lesson we learn from such a case is that some systemic solutions may not be solutions at all. When one of the participants is such an intractable force that he compels the rest of the system to organize around him, excising the organizing entity by blocking the man out and compelling his wife to leave him may seem the best option. In reality, however, such a situation only pushes the problem elsewhere. As therapists we work to make change in systems a process of mutuality. Individuals modify others, and through the recursive loop they are also modified. But not in these intractable cases. We must recognize that there are people who work as catalysts—they enter into a relationship and change the other person, but they do not change themselves. In such cases the therapeutic team, including social service agencies, can work with the homeostatic maintainers within the system and may at times separate the family. However, even if the system is separated, the team should be watchful, cognizant that the man could well move on and repeat the offense elsewhere. If possible, some attempt should be made to do periodic follow-ups to determine the offender's living situation.

ESTABLISHING AND SUSTAINING BOUNDARIES

The concept of boundaries is key in any systemic approach to incest. Incest is not simply a family's private business, it is a delinquent system, one in which extra-firm boundaries must be established by the therapist, if necessary with the help of the law. Part of the strength of family therapy lies in its ability to repair family systems. But incest is one case where such repairs may not be advisable. Establishing boundaries, then, often means violating the cultural expectation that the family be kept together.

The primary problem we address is how to prevent the next incestuous incident. And the therapist who attempts to tame or civilize the incestuous pull while continuing to stress family togetherness may run the risk of sponsoring the next incident by not working sufficiently to sustain boundaries. The work of the therapist who emphasizes keeping the family together may actually prevent people from realizing that in order for them to be sufficient—and safe—they must disengage. In cases of incest establishing protective boundaries should be the first priority. If this can be done with the system kept intact, fine. If not, then the direction should be clear: the therapist must help the family move toward disengagement as quickly as possible, using whatever legal and social resources are available.

UNDERMINING FALSE HOPE

As with violence and other difficult family issues, the therapist treating incest is often confronted by false hope. It is this hope—hope that he won't do it again, hope that things will change—that keeps people in the system. The family hopes that if they do all of the external things, including enlisting outside experts, transformation will come from the outside and change will miraculously occur. But that hope amounts to a denial of the family's own participation in the process of change. The difficult task for the therapist is to encourage the anger and sense of indignation that are absolutely necessary for the motivation of true change. This process, especially the indignation, helps the family to create and maintain boundaries. To bring it about the therapist has to undermine the family's hope that their salvation will come from somewhere or someone outside, or that it will happen automatically just because they have spent time in therapy. Part of the therapist's job is to prepare families for all of the pain and disruption that may be an inescapable part of their process of changing.

TESTING THE SYSTEM

Should one work with the whole family? My friend, Jamshed Morenas, who has had extensive experience consulting in this area for fifteen years, believes that as long as you know that the children are safe then it's important to bring the offender back into the system. He believes that if the offender is expelled the chances of he or she visiting the same behaviors on another community are extremely great. Mr. Morenas, when working with the family, plans a session where he asks the perpetrator what were the specific moments when he started seeing the child, not as a child, but as another adult and potential sexual partner. The hope is that by focusing on these occurrences the other spouse may begin to see his or her role and take some responsibility. This can open the door for working with marital difficulties.

FIRST DO NO HARM

Incest is an area that is rife with controversy. Rigid adherence to any fixed procedure is unwarranted and even dangerous. The interventions must depend on the specifics of the situation such as the age of the child, the intactness of the perpetrator and so forth. Incest is not a homogenous problem.

Clinical Case:
Michele, Struggling to Save Her Marriage

This family, from rural Pennsylvania, was shattered by a profound case of incest between father and daughters. The father had been separated from the family by a social agency, but this separation had not resolved the problems within the system. There remained for this family a kind of glue that bound them together in an unacceptable status quo. They seemed to think that their difficulties could be repaired without the necessity of their facing one another or the disruptive issues that brought about the separation. In fact, it quickly became evident that this family had separated *only* for the sake of the agency and not for themselves. Because the division was imposed from outside, it did not motivate the system to change. Thus, one of the goals of the therapy was to prevent an easy, glib reconciliation.

The job of the consulting therapist in a case like this is to provide the motivation both for genuine separation and for change. To do this one must consider whether the family has the initiative to begin working and must take into account whether the incest was a single incident or chronic and whether it occurred over a long or short period of time. Finally, one must make a preliminary assessment of the abuse of boundaries.

ASSESSMENT USING THE FOUR-DIMENSIONAL MODEL

History

The family consisted of mother, father, and five children. The first four children, two daughters aged fourteen and twelve and two boys aged nine and eight, were the biological children of both parents. The fifth child, a two-year-old daughter, was the result of the mother's involvement with another man during a period when she was separated from her husband. Her husband, the father of the other four children, had agreed to raise this girl as his own.

The father had been having incestuous relations with his two older daughters for the past six years. At the time of the initial session the father was living with his mother. As the family awaited their court date, both parents had been mandated by the court to be in therapy separately. The mother had been participating in a women's therapy group and the father had been involved in both intensive group therapy and individual counseling. The court had allowed the father no contact with the children. He came to this session only with the court's permission, and it was the first time he had seen his wife and children for some months.

Structure

The therapeutic system included the mother, the father, the father's mother, the children, the court, and the therapeutic staff—each parent's therapist and the father's influential perpetrator's group. At the time the family was seen, the parents had a conflictual relationship. At the same time there was inappropriate closeness, for the mother was very protective of the father. There was also overinvolvement between the father and his mother. Needless to say, boundary violations were rife in the system.

Development

The pressures in this system included those brought on by two adolescent children and two more who were nearing adolescence. An additional pressure involved the re-formation of the family, which had been separated, and the formation of joint parenting of the toddler, even though she was the daughter not of the father but of the mother's former lover. In addition, both parents were in their early thirties, and the father was faced with the economic pressure of supporting all of the children, a task made all the more difficult by the fact that he had been incarcerated because of the incest.

Process

There was extreme conflict avoidance in the family, and the mother was seemingly unable to challenge the father. One reason for this, which became apparent during the session, was the father's potential explosiveness. As the session proceeded, the entire therapeutic staff feared increasingly that he would become violent. Indeed, around him one had the sense of sitting on a tinder box; at times I felt he was going to hit me. My subjective experience of this family was that one had to be very careful or one could get hurt. This was not the conflict avoidance of a psychosomatic family, where the people do not wish to hurt one another's feelings because of the fear of abandonment. The conflict avoidance here existed because it was clear that upsetting the father raised a real risk of injury.

THE HOMEOSTATIC MAINTAINER

It became clear that the homeostasis in this family was being maintained by the mother's and the grandmother's unwillingness to challenge the father. Also, the father's therapist saw him as a victim, not as a perpetrator, and thus the man was neither held accountable nor expected to change. Indeed, at points of stress, this therapist would activate to support the father against either his wife or the consultant. I presumed that the therapist was maintaining the same position as the father's mother, who gladly took in her son when he left prison in spite of his sexual abuse of her granddaughters.

The father's therapist was in a particularly difficult position, of course. The theoretical ideology that guided him was individually centered on the father and his plight. Thus it was quite understandable that he identified with the man. But while he was doing his best for his patient, from my position as an outsider I could see that he would support the father at the expense of the children and the wife.

GOALS FOR THE CONSULTANT

As a consultant in the case I had an opportunity to assist in providing brief diagnostic therapy. My aim was to address the fundamental difficulties in the family so that the children would no longer be abused. I saw the key dysfunctional pattern to be avoidance of conflict—the fact that no one ever challenged the father. As a result of remaining unchallenged, the father had never been obliged to be responsible and, indeed, had lived an amoral life, in part because the family allowed it. My diagnostic goal was to support the mother so that she would challenge her husband, in order to see whether he would respond in a responsible way. Whatever his response, this information would be crucial for a prognosis and an eventual recommendation. Moreover, I hoped that the mother might be able to maintain a position of informed mistrust toward her husband and insist on responsible behavior.

As I entered the session my underlying clinical thought was that a family with incest, much like the family described in the following chapter on suicide, presents the most rigid of systems. Whether the family should atomize or work to stay together, the session must be one in which the therapist challenges the flexibility of the system.

THE THERAPY

What follows is a transcription of a family that I saw in consultation for one session. One of the incest victims, the twelve-year-old daughter, was not present at this session; she was away visiting relatives, as were the nine and eight-year-old boys. The family members present were the mother, the father, the oldest daughter (age fourteen) and the father's mother. Also in the room were the mother's and the father's therapists. The two-year-old daughter was in another room.

DR. FISHMAN: How can we help?

FATHER: Yeah, I guess, it's been rough. I guess I growed up in a bad way or something, I don't know. Different things happen in my life. I don't know what I'm really looking for or anything like that. It's been—the past four months—it's been kind of mixed up and everything.

When I begin with the family in an open-ended way, the father classically blames their problems on forces outside his control; he is not responsible. His statement, "I growed up in a bad way," reeks of psycho-babble excuse-making. This response is also consistent with an understandable iatrogenic component that may contribute to the bailing out process. It could easily be a response to therapy he has had since the exposure of the incest, therapy that has focused on the ways in which he was a victim.

The father's response that the family's difficulties—his six years of incest with the daughters—are the result of his having "growed up in a bad way" gives me a clue to the system's homeostatic maintainers that allow this grossly dysfunctional behavior to prevail. Has this been a system where the father was never held responsible for his actions? Was he always bailed out, both figuratively and literally? Were there always people picking up for him? In discussions with the staff on this case I was struck by the grandmother's willingness to take her son in even after learning of his behavior toward his daughters.

DR. FISHMAN (*to the mother*): Michele, what's your perception of this?

MOTHER: My main goal in life is to be able to have a happy family —one marriage for all my life. I knew about my husband's problem when we got married. And I assumed the problem.

DR. FISHMAN: What problem?

MOTHER: The abuse that he had when he was a child. (*To her husband:*) I tried to help you with what you were going through then and leave it in the past. (*To the therapist:*) I feel somehow that I failed in some ways in helping him to overcome this. I feel like everything I ever wanted is just falling apart right now.

DR. FISHMAN: Is it pretty hopeless, do you think?

MOTHER: I don't know about hopeless—I always have hope.

DR. FISHMAN: How old are your kids?

MOTHER: The oldest is fourteen tomorrow, that's Diane. Debbie, who's not with us today, is twelve. Jason is nine, Mark is eight, and Mary-Lou is two.

It is clearer now that the mother is one of the people who is helping this man escape responsibility. By implying that his abuse of their daughters is a result of his being abused as a child, she provides yet another context in which he is not responsible for his actions. In this system the locus of control is placed not within the man but somehow in the principal characters who abused him in his childhood. The net effect is a system organized around allowing this man to remain an ethically irresponsible preadolescent.

DR. FISHMAN (*after a long pause*): You've been in therapy?

MOTHER: In group therapy. I started individually but the hours I could get were just too inconvenient, so I stopped.

FATHER: We both go to school.

DR. FISHMAN: What are you studying?

FATHER:	She's studying to be a nurse's aid, and I'm going to trade school to become a plumber.
DR. FISHMAN:	How's it going?
FATHER:	Oh, pretty good, I guess.
DR. FISHMAN:	I'm not convinced.
FATHER:	Pardon me?
DR. FISHMAN:	I'm not convinced.
FATHER:	Well, I can't keep up sometimes—when a lot of times you have a lot of things on your mind and everything. I just try to do my best.
DR. FISHMAN *(to the father)*:	Are you going to finish?
FATHER:	I'm going to try.
DR. FISHMAN *(to the mother)*:	Is he going to finish?
MOTHER:	He is going to finish.
FATHER:	Yeah. When I do something I usually finish it.
MOTHER:	I very rarely know him to start something that he hasn't finished.
DR. FISHMAN:	That's been part of the problem all these years. You're studying to be a nurse's aid?
MOTHER:	And learn home care.
DR. FISHMAN *(to the father)*:	Is she going to finish?
FATHER:	Oh, yeah.
DR. FISHMAN:	No question about her finishing?
FATHER:	No question. I supported her for fifteen years—now she's gonna finish so she can support me for fifteen years. (*The mother and father both laugh.*)

This immature father has fantasies of being financially mothered by his wife, who in many ways is already his emotional mother.

DR. FISHMAN:	So what are some of the problems that you have as a couple?
MOTHER:	As a couple?
FATHER:	Kids. We fight about kids all the time. Well, not all the time, but most.
DR. FISHMAN:	In what way?
FATHER:	Punishments.

MOTHER: He thinks I'm too lenient, and I think he's too strict. When we argue I tend to give in at one time and he'll give in at another. He's just the type that when he gets mad, he says what's on his mind, and then he's not upset anymore. I'm the type that when I get mad I like a good argument and to talk it all out—even if I have to scream and yell. But he doesn't ever give me that chance to let all that out before he wants to make up.

DR. FISHMAN: So nothing ever gets resolved.

MOTHER: No. So then he says it's the same old crap all the time. Then he wonders why I argue about the same old crap every time. It's because I never feel I get anything resolved.

This lack of resolution is significant in terms of the presenting problem. To the extent that problems are not resolved, the vulnerable couple becomes increasingly distant as time goes on, and the symmetrical, yet underground, battle ensues. This battle makes it more likely that the growing schizmogenesis will be stabilized by the participation of a third party. According to some family therapy theorists, at this point the child is recruited by the father or offered by the mother to compensate for affectional deficits in the spousal subsystem. However, there are problems with this theory: it has no limits, and in some cases it can expand into precisely the myth that "if my wife gave herself to me I wouldn't take from the child." To accept this myth would lead to an undoing of the therapeutic possibilities and would endanger the child. When approaching incest problems, it is not simply a matter of repairing the affectional exchanges between the adults in order to protect the child. That orientation can jeopardize the whole system, particularly the victimized child.

For this couple the most severe difficulties seem to involve the area of sex. But these problems are never addressed to the point of resolution. Indeed they will have to be raised somewhere along the line as a central issue in the therapy. But in a family such as this, where the presenting problem is so destructive, the protection of the children is the issue that must be addressed first. As the session continues, it is becoming increasingly clear to me that the mother does not see the children as a priority. She seems to think that the couple is more important than the children. The immediate question, then, becomes whether the children will be safe if this family stays together.

DR. FISHMAN: The question I have, from what I heard about your story, is why you would want to be together. I wonder why you would take him back. As a mother, you need to protect your children. That's more important than being a couple.

MOTHER: Um-hm. My kids complain. But I still love him, so . . .

DR. FISHMAN: That's a problem. Don't worry, you'll get over that. I think that you really need to think about that very seriously. Can you trust him? See, what troubles me is that when I asked, "What is the problem?" Walt said (*pausing and turning to the father*) that the problem is that he grew up in a bad way. He is not taking responsibility. He's not saying "I did something wrong" but "I grew up in a bad way."

FATHER: What makes you say that I did something wrong?

DR. FISHMAN: That's what I'm talking about. It's exactly what I'm talking about. Talk with—you call him your husband at this point?

MOTHER: Um-hm.

DR. FISHMAN: Talk with Walt about that in terms of responsibility.

FATHER: I don't understand what you're saying.

DR. FISHMAN: You understand—the incest.

This intervention illustrates important principles for working with incestuous families. The mother's priorities should be first to shelter and protect the child and then to think about the marriage. The therapist's primary job is to keep the children safe and not allow the mother to be brutalized. To achieve this the therapist must give priority to maintaining a strong boundary between the family and the father.

Initially the father tells how he is trying to get himself together, and I show him respect for that. But more revealing is his question, "What makes you say that I did something wrong?" I use this interchange to show the mother that her husband does not take responsibility for his actions and that without taking responsibility there will be no change in his behavior. This represents a challenge to the mother that I hope will lead her to take the initiative and come to the realization that it is indeed *her* responsibility to make the decision whether or not to take her husband back. The therapist's goal here is to reinforce the understanding that the ultimate responsibility resides in the contemporary relationships within the family, not in the parents' past or in the workings of the legal system.

MOTHER: In other words, what you're saying is that he isn't accepting the fact that, as an adult, he is responsible for the way he is now. Is that correct?

DR. FISHMAN: [For] what has transpired.

MOTHER: Then he's responsible for what's happened since he was a kid.

DR. FISHMAN (to the father):   How old are you now?

FATHER: Thirty-four.

DR. FISHMAN (to the mother):   Why don't you talk about truth?

MOTHER: How I feel about it?

DR. FISHMAN: Whether Walt accepts responsibility for that.

FATHER: What I've done now, yeah. But from the way you stated it that I did something wrong when I was a kid and I have to take responsibility for it, that's what I was looking at. And I don't see where I did something wrong when I was a kid.

DR. FISHMAN: I agree with you there. It has nothing to do with it. I'm agreeing 100 percent. What's occurred over the last six or seven years has nothing to do with your childhood.

FATHER: No, no, what I'm saying is . . .

DR. FISHMAN: Or anything that you had done as a child.

FATHER: What I'm saying is that when you said that when I was a kid I did something wrong and I got to accept the facts about it, I thought you were talking about what I did as a kid. . . . But now, yeah. We've already talked about that, and sure I made mistakes.

Of course, the father may be telling the truth: he may have defensively perceived the inquiry as pertaining to what had happened in childhood and considered it unbelievable that he should accept blame for those distant events. If that is the case, however, his tendency to disassociate from the present would be even more reason to focus on the prevention of a quick patching up of relations between him and his wife.

DR. FISHMAN: See, Michele, when you bring up the fact that you can't seem to address conflicts and get anything resolved, that worries me in terms of your future as a family. There will be things that come up. Why don't you take something, take some issue and see if you can resolve it.

MOTHER: Take any issue?

DR. FISHMAN: Any issue that is important to you that you feel hasn't been resolved. Because if you can resolve things that way, it's a better indication that you will be able to work things out.

My focus here is on the principle that in dealing with issues like incest one cannot prove a negative. Instead one has to see dysfunctional patterns resolved in the treatment room.

MOTHER (*to the father*): Well, one of the things that bothers me a lot is the fact that you're not as close to the older two kids as you are to the younger three. In terms of affection and showing that you care.

FATHER (*first pausing*): I don't know why that is.

DR. FISHMAN: I would deal with a more difficult issue. Is there an issue in terms of the two of you, not something that involves the kids? (*He pauses.*) The issue about how you deal with the kids is something that can be dealt with over a longer period of time. But in terms of you two as a couple . . .

MOTHER: There's not too many issues just between the two of us. Not resolving an argument that we started . . .

DR. FISHMAN: What's the last argument you had?

I am searching for a concrete issue the couple could discuss, an issue that they both have strong feelings about and one from which intensity might be generated.

FATHER: Don't know.

MOTHER: He says I don't want to—you know—he says I never come to him. I've tried, but it's hard for me. I've never been a very aggressive person. You know, we've been together for fifteen years. I've felt that I've often shown it. . . .

DR. FISHMAN (*to the father*): Do you feel that Michele is there for you emotionally?

FATHER: I feel she's there for me in a lot of things—emotional support and. . . .

DR. FISHMAN: Is there any way that she's not there for you? Or is everything just perfect?

FATHER: No. She's been there, she's been my backbone through everything. She's helped me through fifteen years. She's helped me through other things. She's been there.

DR. FISHMAN: Are there ways in which Walt isn't there for you?

MOTHER: Well, the only thing—I'm a very sensitive person and I know that sometimes I let that rule me. When I think that he is not trying to get closer with her [their daughter, Diane], it hurts me a lot. I think Diane is at an age when she needs to be close to her daddy, and to be able to do things with him.

My jaw drops open. I am increasingly concerned that mother is so anxious to have father more involved with his elder daughters. I can't help but wonder about mother's part in this incest. For the present, I chose to ignore this and focus on issues that will facilitate my joining with mother.

If the couple could resolve an important issue right there in the room, that would be an indication that they could resolve similar problems on the outside. Furthermore, the work in the therapy room could provide a template for a new way of interfacing. Of course, if they could not work on and resolve a representative issue with the help of the therapist, it would not bode well for their success in addressing the problems they were confronted with in their family life. More important, if they could not effectively resolve their difficulties and become closer, then we could not be assured that the system would not continue to victimize and exploit the children.

In the next segment we begin dealing with the essential question of responsibility in protecting the children. There was a dramatic backdrop to this segment. The youngest child was in the next room. The doors were somewhat flimsy and the child could hear the parents. As the tension increased, the child in the other room began to cry more and more loudly, eventually becoming so upset that I suggested the mother bring her into the room.

To let this child suffer in the other room while we are talking about protecting children would have belied our message of the importance of caring for children.

DR. FISHMAN: You really want to know whether he's changing or not because of the kids. So really, we shouldn't get away from that. But why would you want to take him back, what would need to change so that you would take him back?

MOTHER: Well, I would want him to get therapy too.

DR. FISHMAN: Therapy is great, but how will he have to change?

MOTHER: How would he have to change?

DR. FISHMAN: Why don't you talk to Walt. Are you interested in having him back?

MOTHER: Yeah, very much.

DR. FISHMAN: Maybe you could get somebody else?

MOTHER: Well, my kids love their dad.

DR. FISHMAN: But that's not a reason to stay with somebody.

There is no doubt that I am expressing my own bias and convictions here. I feel that the family's values are distorted. The mother's protection of her husband and the desire to keep the couple intact has been allowed to override the needs of the offspring.

MOTHER: I love him. He's always been there in every way for support, he's genuinely a loving man.

DR. FISHMAN: Well, yes, we know that. With all due respect, I wonder what he would have to do so you would trust him.

MOTHER: I don't completely trust him, I have that doubt in the back of my mind.

DR. FISHMAN: Are you one of these women who is just kind of a pushover? (*To the father:*) Is she really a pushover?

FATHER: In some ways.

DR. FISHMAN: Is she? See, I don't think your kids can afford it.

MOTHER: Well, I'll be very protective of my children. First of all, he knows that I always made that important from the time I had my children.

FATHER: That's something I would never do again.

MOTHER: But I will always have that doubt. I don't know if I would ever tell you when the kids were home, I wouldn't get over that doubt. It would probably be years ... but I would have to be very protective for a long time. I would like for you to accept or find the true meaning of fatherhood, what it means, the truth, responsibilities.

DR. FISHMAN: In other words, if Walt were to do that you'd have a sense that he was really being a father and not a playmate.

MOTHER: Well, not completely.

DR. FISHMAN: But you'd have a sense?

MOTHER: I would have a sense that he would at least be trying to accomplish that role.

DR. FISHMAN: Why don't you talk to him about it.

MOTHER: What would you be willing to do to find this? To find out what the role is?

FATHER: I've been there.

MOTHER: Then search it to find out.

FATHER: So, you know I'm seeing all these people to find out where i went wrong. My life is all in a shambles because of it.

DR. FISHMAN: Hold on one second, because I think this is a point in which you (*turning to the mother*) get quiet and get soft and don't push it.

MOTHER: I don't have the courage.

DR. FISHMAN: Is that an acceptable answer?

In the following sequence it is clear that the mother pathetically believes that she can hold on to her husband and that somehow some outside force will cause him to be responsible. She remains convinced that fatherhood can be taught, even when her husband disagrees. The motivation to change is not generated from within. The father does not have the initiative to change.

MOTHER: I need to know if he is willing to follow through with it. Take courses or whatever.

FATHER: To what?

MOTHER: If they suggest that you take courses or something would you be willing to follow through with it?

FATHER: You can't take a course on how to be a father. All they can do is tell you what it's like to be a father. But you can't go by what they say. A father isn't just made by a book.

MOTHER: What about guidelines?

FATHER: Sure you can have guidelines. But you can't always follow all the guidelines.

MOTHER: Then it would be—probably something would cause you to lose control, and . . .

FATHER: That's why I'm going to therapy.

MOTHER: That doesn't always specify what it is you would need to help you with your problem.

FATHER: I don't see what you're saying.

MOTHER: Okay, you've been going to therapy, and one of the things you have to work on is to control your impulses.

FATHER: Right.

MOTHER: But there aren't any rules or anything for your impulses—that they can give you to do to help you control them.

FATHER: How can you tell—from just the little time we're together?

MOTHER: Well—I've seen the rules that they have for you to graduate. But I haven't seen anything to help you with any problems.

The mother is looking for outside rules to impose control on her husband.

As the sequence progresses she talks with her husband about having sex with their daughter as if it is simply one more area of infraction, like having too much to drink. Thus the incest is declared to be one more forgivable area. It is increasingly apparent that these parents do not at all recognize the enormity of the father's infraction.

FATHER: I see what you're saying—about our sex, when I get horny I'm supposed to control it.

MOTHER: No, I'm not just saying our sex, I'm saying when you get impulses for, like, when you want to have sex with my daughter.

FATHER: How can you tell?

MOTHER: I'm saying if they did give you them—would you follow by those rules?

FATHER: First, you're asking me what you ain't seen—then you're asking me would I.

MOTHER: Well, if they had.

FATHER: Of course I would.

MOTHER: Because I don't know if they do that.

FATHER: There's two different things: the impulse with the kids or impulse with you is two different things. So I follow my impulses with you a lot different than I follow my impulses with the kids. So you only seen the one I follow for you.

MOTHER: Okay.

At this point I was looking at this system in awe, asking myself if this woman indeed knew what was "okay." The triviality assigned to the incest is extremely inappropriate and indicates strongly that there is danger ahead.

DR. FISHMAN:	So what about the impulses? That's very important. What about the impulses between the two of you?
FATHER:	When I feel my impulses, what I want to do is between me and her.
DR. FISHMAN:	Talk about that.
FATHER:	She don't follow the impulses between me and her. It's always later, or she's always put off.
MOTHER:	That's true.

The father's statement is an indication of the survival of the repression or deflection theory: if he did not have to repress his sexual impulses with his wife, he would not need to abuse his daughter. This theory of repression and deflection may have been the basis of this family's past therapy. The father's therapist felt that somehow the father's abuse of his daughter was at least understandable, if not justified, because of the insufficiencies between the husband and wife, and he assumed that a therapy designed to repair the marital relationship would cause the incest to cease. This assumption was dangerous. In most therapy, even with very difficult cases, we can assume that the generational boundaries will hold, but such assumptions are shattered in cases of incest. It was, in fact, quite possible that this man would continue to use both his wife and his daughters. The abuse of the children was very likely independent of the availability of the spouse.

DR. FISHMAN:	The question is, can you trust Walt not to go out of control?
FATHER:	I don't go out of control.
MOTHER:	What do you mean by out of control?
DR. FISHMAN:	Get very angry—lose his temper—or have sex with your daughters.
MOTHER:	Oh, yes.
FATHER:	There's one thing, I would not hit nobody.
DR. FISHMAN:	You hit the wall.
FATHER:	I've hit a wall, I'll hit anything but I won't hit anybody.

DR. FISHMAN: You see what you're doing is very important, you're being very clear in terms of what you need from Walt. Are there other needs? See, it's your responsibility, it has to be. Are there ways in which you will be able to spend some time . . . the two of you and one of your children? Will you be able to see what kind of father Walt is? Maybe Walt can help you with that.

MOTHER: I would love to be able to take just one of the children and spend some time together with Walt. One idea would be to take one full day with one child and to see his type of reaction with that child and [*to her husband*] the different reaction you have with each child.

FATHER: We got too much things going, we ain't got enough time to spend the day.

MOTHER: No, I'm saying if we had the time to take one whole day with each child, even if it's just one Saturday a week and take that with one child and the following Saturday with another child. We don't have to have money to go and do that, just take a picnic, that's all.

FATHER: We get there, I'll go to sleep.

MOTHER: Unless it's the baby, because she makes you play with her.

DR. FISHMAN: See, I think that's giving you information. Giving you information that maybe you shouldn't be together.

FATHER: No, it's just that I work Friday nights.

DR. FISHMAN: I don't mean just about the specifics, but I think you need to think as the mother: "That's information."

The tension in the room was beginning to build. The father was getting angrier and angrier. We had arrived at an issue that crystalized the problem in the system: can this man be a nurturing, caring father, or is he instead a man who is going to abuse his children? He had not, after all, had a relationship where he acted like a true parent. If the mother and father could be together with the children in a way that allowed him to work on becoming a true parent figure, then both the therapeutic system and the mother would have an indication that he could indeed function in a different way.

It should also be noted that there was a complementary aspect of this family system: in some ways the mother acted to exclude her husband and so contributed to his inability to function as a true father figure. As a result he felt treated as only a breadwinner, responsible for supporting five children and a demanding wife. Nevertheless, a characteristic pattern in this man's life was that he organized the surrounding systems so that they accommodated to him. At this moment, however, his wife, with the therapist's support, was asking him to do the accommodating. This situation could be used as a diagnostic test: if he does not accommodate here, he cannot be expected to accommodate to the generational and societal boundaries that would restrain him from abusing his children whenever he has the urge.

> MOTHER: What would you do if you didn't have to work all the time? What would you do then?
> FATHER: I would be able to sleep at night on Friday and Saturday nights.
> MOTHER: What would you do during the day?
> FATHER: Catch up on everything else I had to do prior in the week. You know there's a lot of things I have to do. Keep the van running.
> MOTHER: Take the day off. That's all I'm asking, just take the day off.
> FATHER: That means twice as much work I got to do the following day.

I suspect that this man stayed with his cars and vans so that he would not have to get close to people. Creating this artificial boundary may have been the best he could do to protect the world a little bit from himself. As the mother continued to try to get him to spend some time with her and the children, his responses revealed that he was not comfortable in his relationship with his wife and children.

> MOTHER: Well what you're saying is that the kids don't come first anymore.
> FATHER: What do you think I'm out there working for? Why do you think I'm out there keeping the van running so you can take them to the doctors if you have to, in case of an emergency or something like that?
> MOTHER: Don't worry about the kids, because they're growing and the things that they need, they're the emotional needs.
> FATHER: I never got them.
> MOTHER: Well, that doesn't mean you have to deprive the children.
> FATHER: I don't know what it's like, okay. I grew up where I had to take care of myself.
> MOTHER: But you should know how hard it was as a kid.

DR. FISHMAN:	The thing is, do you want the kids not to get what you didn't get?
FATHER:	No, I want the kids to get it. I want the kids to learn affection.
MOTHER:	But you want it to be from me, and not from you.
FATHER:	I got something in me that's hard.

As the father says "I got something in me that's hard," an honest description of his affective limitations, he glances across the room at his therapist. Apparently they had had many sessions on this issue, sessions in which the father may have somehow felt that his own lack of nurturing as a child somehow justified his abuse of his own children. In glancing at his therapist he seems almost to be looking for protection. As the session continues I have a sense that the father and his therapist are joined in a "helpful" stance. They are in a coalition.

MOTHER:	I know.
FATHER:	Like something that was put there a long time ago.

Observing the father's intractability and his seemingly impermeable defense of "something in me that's hard," I attempt to bolster the wife's position by using her as my co-therapist. As the challenging consultant I increase the intensity by bringing in the larger context, asking the mother whether she is seeing anyone else.

DR. FISHMAN:	Are you dating at this point?
MOTHER:	No.
DR. FISHMAN:	Are you legally separated?
MOTHER:	No.
DR. FISHMAN:	You're not legally separated. Did you think about it?
MOTHER:	No.
FATHER:	I love her too much.
MOTHER (*to Dr. Fishman*):	Well, don't you think that's the reason.
FATHER:	What do you think I'm doing? I'm going to these people to get help and you're pushing all the shit on me at once.
DR. FISHMAN:	So you believe that the helpers are going to change things for you and the family. We as helpers are terrific, and we help lots of people. But we don't do much.

FATHER: No, I don't believe you guys are going to help us change. You're going to help us, but in a certain way.

DR. FISHMAN: All the helpers that you had really didn't make much difference. I think you have to believe if you're going to change.

FATHER: How can you have a family separated and be able to live a normal life and then turn around and do what people suggest you do?

The father is working hard to have the agency people turn him loose to go back to his family. I am reluctant to do so, but I sense that he might be effective in turning around the various helpers so that they would endorse his quick return to the family. I feel that a premature return is potentially disastrous and attempt to instill the thought that any return must be done with great caution.

DR. FISHMAN: You see, your wife just said very clearly that you had hope. She hopes that you have hope. She is making it a kind of laboratory to see if maybe you have a day that's just for your family.

FATHER: That's what I'm hoping for.

DR. FISHMAN: But with all due respect, your feet don't follow your words.

I was struggling with the battle for initiative. This family thought that their changing would in some way be done for them by their professional helpers: since they had elicited so much help, they would be magically transformed and their problems would be ameliorated. This notion of powerful outside help allowed them to justify not doing very much work themselves. This was one homeostatic force. Another was the persistent hope expressed by the mother. This hope, fostered by the legion of therapists, kept them in there struggling, but it was essential to convey the reality that their only hope lay in taking responsibility for their problems and making immediate change in this very enactment.

DR. FISHMAN *(to the mother)*:   Are you going to continue your therapy? Do you think that's a right move?

MOTHER: I think it's worthwhile.

DR. FISHMAN: Do you think you learn from it?

MOTHER: I think that will eventually come.

DR. FISHMAN:	You are hoping that the other situation will change, aren't you?
MOTHER:	What situation?
DR. FISHMAN:	The one that you were referring to earlier—the illegal behavior—the incest.
MOTHER:	Uh-huh.
DR. FISHMAN:	Didn't your hope keep you from doing anything?
MOTHER:	What do you mean?

The mother's reaction here is the symmetrical equivalent of the father's earlier reaction, when he did not understand what he had done wrong. Tending toward quick healing and denial, she glosses over the atrocity her daughters have experienced, thereby making its repetition likely.

DR. FISHMAN:	Did you hope that his behavior would stop—that he would change his behavior?
MOTHER:	What behavior?
DR. FISHMAN:	With your daughters.
MOTHER:	Yeah.
DR. FISHMAN:	You believe in hope.
MOTHER:	Yeah.
DR. FISHMAN:	I don't believe in hope. You know why? Because to the extent that people believe in hope they don't change. I'm going to step out now for a minute. But I have a clear sense that he's already told you what you want to know.
FATHER:	I ain't told nothing.

The father is getting more and more angry as he accurately perceives my intent, and I am afraid that he is going to lean over and hit me. I am slowing down the forces that would return him to the family, and he does not like it.

DR. FISHMAN:	You'd be surprised.

At this point I was the lone skeptic in the room. This was the hardest part of my job in this session—being the voice of hopelessness. I leave the room and go behind the mirror. As I leave, the father's therapist moves into the seat next to the father and starts talking to him.

In the sequence that follows it is quite clear that the father did read my intentions correctly and that he would try to defy me by being more truthful.

THERAPIST:	Why are you so upset?
FATHER:	He was trying to get her separated from me. That's wrong.
THERAPIST:	The impression that I got was that the situation was not going to change, that hope is not going to change it.
FATHER:	Everybody has hope. He said he doesn't believe in hope. That doesn't make any difference. But when he made that remark about "your feet don't follow your words," that got me upset.
THERAPIST:	That was your impression.
FATHER:	I'm going to prove him wrong.
THERAPIST:	What did you feel about it?
FATHER:	I feel he's working against us.
THERAPIST:	At what point did you feel that?
FATHER:	As soon as he said that.
THERAPIST (*to the mother*):	How about you, did you feel that?
MOTHER:	Well, I have doubts about me and Walt living together. I don't know if we can do that—if I would be a good mother.

The mother's doubts about their living together and about her capacity to mother correctly are a change from her earlier glib confidence, apparently endorsed by the helpers, that it was just a matter of one more round.

(Upon returning to the room I am relieved not to be seated next to father any more and to have a six-foot three-inch tall therapist between the two of us. As I return, the father's therapist offers to give me back the seat next to the father. I indicate that he should stay put!)

FATHER:	I have a feeling your idea that you're not a good mother may come from . . .
THERAPIST:	From what?
FATHER:	From—something, what?
MOTHER:	From the feeling that I'm not protecting my children.
DR. FISHMAN:	No, you're not. You weren't . . .
MOTHER:	That makes me feel like I let it happen.
DR. FISHMAN:	Partly you did.

MOTHER: I had no idea what was going on.

DR. FISHMAN: The question now is, can you trust him.

MOTHER: I don't know if I can trust him yet.

DR. FISHMAN: You see, what we did earlier, we said if you could spend a day together, if somehow Walt would arrange his schedule, it would give you a sense that he could change his behavior and his impulses, or whatever, for you and for the kids. So far, what I've heard is that he said "no."

One of the forces that had allowed the mother to be blind for so long to her daughters' abuse was the fact that she shared a patriarchal notion that men can do no wrong. She believed that her role was to make up for her husband's damaged childhood and to exonerate him. Her devalued self-concept as a woman was part of what permitted her to accept the abuse of her girls. As she suddenly began to realize that she may, in a complementary way, have been involved in the incest, she became defensive. I needed to enlist her support, not alienate her, so her defensive response was a clear indication that I should backtrack.

MOTHER: I feel like I'm being contradicted, because I go to group therapy and they tell me that it's not my fault that it happened, that I had no idea what was going on.

DR. FISHMAN: It's certainly not.

MOTHER: But in here it's my fault because I let it happen.

DR. FISHMAN: I don't think that's correct. I hope you're not getting that. What I'm asking is how you can keep things from happening in the future. How can you look at him and trust him?

The mother has, of course, caught me in a contradiction. As she begins to acknowledge her role in the incest, the danger is that she may drop totally into depression and self-blame. I try to avert this and to get her to think about what to do next.

MOTHER: I don't know, it's going to take a lot of time, with a lot of safety precautions—things like that.

DR. FISHMAN: Okay, that's true. My question is, from what I've heard, Walt says he will not accommodate to you.

FATHER: That's not what I'm saying.

MOTHER: I don't believe that that's . . .

DR. FISHMAN: Well, then, talk to him. Maybe I'm wrong.

FATHER: My kids come first, but who is going to put food, clothes, and whatever they need on their backs?

DR. FISHMAN
(looking at the
mother):

FATHER: You don't have to convince me.

FATHER: I got to, she knows; I have to take care of business around the house and do what I have to do to get a little extra money while I'm going to school.

MOTHER: Okay, let me give you a "for instance," okay?

FATHER: No "for instance."

MOTHER: Yeah, just this.

FATHER: No "for instance," because you can't do it right now.

MOTHER: Will you just listen to me, please. You graduate in December and I graduate in September, all right?

FATHER: When we get on our feet . . .

MOTHER: Will you listen . . .

FATHER: When we get on our feet and I can take Saturdays and Sundays off and not have to worry about time and we can both take the baby or whatever . . .

MOTHER: I know it's hard right now . . .

FATHER: But I'm not looking for when we get on our feet, I'm looking for tomorrow, the next day.

MOTHER: It's going to take time anyway. I know that.

FATHER: I don't look for the future, I look for tomorrow.

MOTHER: I look for the future.

FATHER: I don't and you know that.

MOTHER: Well, I have to look for the future because my kids are going to be there.

FATHER: I might be killed tomorrow, you never know.

MOTHER: But still you have to look. You're the one who always told me that—before you changed.

FATHER: I never told you that.

MOTHER: Yeah, you always took out life insurance policies and everything else.

FATHER: No.

MOTHER: You said you wanted to make sure the kids and I were taken care of.

DR. FISHMAN: See what's happened? You said that you never really resolved anything and you never have a sense of satisfaction in terms of issues. You started an issue, and now somehow you're talking about life insurance.

MOTHER: I was talking about looking into the future.

DR. FISHMAN: Something very practical.

MOTHER: And, I was just saying for instance when we get on our feet and we can start seeing each other with the children, it really won't be an issue whether the kids need this or that.

DR. FISHMAN *(to the mother)*: Do you have a sense that you're backing down? That you're doing what everybody does with this man? They accommodate to him: he doesn't budge. If he says he can't spend one evening with you and the kids, he's so busy, but you're saying now that it's the future, isn't that backing down?

MOTHER: I know what he's saying isn't what he's saying because I know if he has the time he will spend time with us.

DR. FISHMAN: Time is a funny thing. We make time for what we have to do. You said that yourself.

FATHER: Right, make time for what we have to do, and when I got to work on the van or I have to work in the yard, I have to make time for them, sure. I'd like to make time for a lot of things, but . . .

DR. FISHMAN: You don't have to convince me, you have to convince Michele whether she will be able to trust you.

FATHER: After fifteen years of marriage if she can't trust me, well, I can't say that. There is no real way that she can say that she can trust me.

DR. FISHMAN: Don't be so optimistic.

FATHER: And there ain't no real way that I can trust her. It's her word and it's my word, that's it.

DR. FISHMAN: Do you believe him?

MOTHER: I know what he is saying is true, he trusted my word. Do you want to go play with the kids, huh? You tired? Do you think you will ever have time for the kids?

FATHER: Yeah.

MOTHER: When it's convenient. Would you make time?

FATHER: It's hard to say.

MOTHER: I make time after the housework. I make time. You don't think the yard could wait one day. There's a lot of times we can just do things together; we all used to pitch in and do the yard together, do the house together. That would be a way of spending time together.

The mother further accommodates to her husband by saying that they can be together while doing various chores around the house. This offer allows him to continue to resist extending himself any further.

DR. FISHMAN: I see clearly that you're a very caring mother. You make tremendous sacrifices for those kids.

In the hope of keeping the mother from backing off, I move to support her.

FATHER: I suppose I don't?

DR. FISHMAN   Okay, we need to think about whether you want to do
(*to the thera-*   therapy with this couple right now. I don't know if there's
pist):   hope, I don't know if it's worth it. (*To the couple:*) With all due respect, maybe you could do better not being together. (*To the mother:*) How old are you?

MOTHER: Thirty-one.

DR. FISHMAN: A young woman.

FATHER (*to*   And you're a real fucking asshole too.
Dr. Fishman):

DR. FISHMAN: You don't prove anything by a hassle with me.

FATHER: That's the way I feel. I come here to try to get something done and to work together with my wife and you sit here.

DR. FISHMAN: I'm trying to be responsible, responsible to you as a family.

THERAPIST (*to*   Don't let those feelings stay inside. It's important to work
the father):   them through.

The father and his therapist both turn in their chairs, the therapist turning away from me. The father is crying and the therapist is also crying, wiping the corners of his eyes. The father, who has just showered me with expletives, is obviously very angry. A clear sense of a homeostatic maintainer in operation can be seen in the therapist's telling this man, whose difficulty has been a lack of impulse control, to express his feelings fully. I must confess to having some personal concern here as well; if the therapist continues to encourage the father to express himself, I could be in trouble.

FATHER: I ain't giving up what I have for you or nobody.
DR. FISHMAN: You just talk to your wife, and I think your wife will be very happy to take you. But the question is whether you can change, too. See, it's pretty simple. All your wife says is that she wants to spend an evening with you and the kids. Okay, I'm going to leave it to you. You know, I was impressed with the work that you're doing and how well you're proceeding, and I respect that you're starting a new career. The question is, do the two of you want to start a new relationship?
MOTHER: Better than what we had before.
DR. FISHMAN: Yes.
MOTHER: We can't keep the one we had.

Summary

The primary goal of this session was to see that the incest was not repeated. Great intensity was generated in the hope of producing an essential realization in the mother that whether or not she had any responsibility for the original incest, she indeed had a responsibility to see that it did not recur. Our job was to protect the children from being traumatized and victimized any further. That meant that our goal was not to keep the family together but to transform the system so that the children would be protected and all family members would be able to differentiate, feel safe, and get on with their lives. As part of the therapy it became necessary to utilize the law to create a boundary between the children and the father, limiting and controlling his access to them. Furthermore, the boundaries had to make very clear the difference between the parental functions and the spousal functions. Our task was aimed at creating a vertical, generational boundary instead of a horizontal boundary between father and child. This boundary-making had to be done in the mother's presence, for reasons of safety, because the mother in many ways was the key to effective control of the father's access to the children.

The session raised some very important theoretical concerns. Why did the father get so angry? Was it because he thought I was expelling him from the family? Did he sense a coalition against him, a coalition that reminded him of experiences at home? Was he angry because I was provoking his wife to drop him? Let us consider the sequence of events. I began by generating considerable intensity around the issue of his spending some time with his wife and one of the children. The man refused, saying he had to take care of a van for the family. The mother, remaining adamant, replied, "All I want is to spend a little time together." Still he refused. Why? Could it be that he was, perhaps understandably, engaged with his therapist in a process of building walls, and that I was beginning to dismantle that process? The man did say that he very much wanted to be with his family and to move back home. It is possible that he wanted walls built because without them he was afraid he might slip. Because of this understandable fear I scaled down the suggested amount of time to be spent with his wife and child, limiting it to just an evening. Even this, however, proved too much of an accommodation for this man.

Whatever theoretical insight we might gain into the father's behavior, the quality of the system suggested that the man was fundamentally unaccustomed to accommodating to others. Instead he insisted that everyone else accommodate to him. I saw this immobility as a very grave prognostic sign. For if this father would not adapt to a small change when he had so much to gain, what hope was there of his adapting to control his impulsive desires if he should get back together with his family?

As a result of the father's intractability, I had few illusions about this family's capacity to transform itself on its own. It would be up to the external societal system to remain responsible and vigilant and to accept a constant role in the monitoring of rules and in the maintenance of boundaries. With this family there was simply not enough responsibility and initiative for self-directed change. In this case we had at the center an extraordinary prince, a narcissist, who organized the family system around his needs. As long as this was true, a continuation of the incest would be possible and the daughters would remain in jeopardy.

7

The Suicidal Adolescent: A Stranger in Paradox

> He believed that death was a sign that you were ready to further your knowledge to travel higher, learning and understanding more as you went. . . . He was a dreamer, a believer, a competitor and most of all he was a striver. He strove for what he wanted until the day he died.
>
> —A seventeen-year-old boy who killed himself
> a short time after writing his
> own eulogy as a school assignment

OVER THE PAST DECADE suicide among youths has emerged as a national epidemic, the second leading cause of death (after accidents) for American teenagers and young adults. Each year suicide claims more than five thousand Americans between the ages of fifteen and twenty-four. The growth in this phenomenon is truly alarming. Since 1950 the youth suicide rate has almost tripled, from 4.8 per 100,000 youths to 12.5 per 100,000 in 1985 (Drake 1987).

Despite the statistical data there has been surprisingly little research that deals specifically with adolescent suicide (McKenry, Tishler, and Kelley 1982; Drake 1987). Those who have studied the phenomenon list a number of possible precipitating or contributing factors, such as introjected anger (Durkheim 1951), social isolation (Trout 1980), alienation from peers (Barter, Swayback, and Todd 1968), and drug and alcohol abuse (Tishler, McKenry, and Morgan 1981). The necessary element in all adolescent suicide attempts is depression, although it is not by itself sufficient. Whether the depression is overtly manifest or is masked by another problem or by denial (Carlson 1981), the connection between depression and suicide is well supported (Rosenblatt 1981; Cassoria 1979; Mattsson, Seese, and Hawkins 1969).

Regardless of how one determines the cause, the therapeutic approach advocated in these pages remains the same: we must look at depression and the ensuing suicidal behavior as emanating from a dysfunctional social context and view the social ecology as both the problem and the solution. Understanding the context that leads to suicidal depression allows us to transform the ecology and to free the members of the system from the trap of hopeless desperation.

THE IMPORTANCE OF THE FAMILY

The research that is available suggests that difficulties in the family are the most important predictor of adolescent suicide. For example, Joseph Teicher and Jerry Jacobs (1966) see suicidal adolescents as having poor parent-child relationships and family conflict which preclude the supportive relationships and successful modeling that would allow the youth to cope with the problems and stress associated with adolescence. Christopher Williams and Christina Lyons (1976) cite clinical studies indicating a relationship between a disorganized nuclear family and adolescent suicide attempts. A survey of the literature by Sue Petzel and Mary Riddle (1981) further supports the finding that suicidal youths experience greater family disorganization than do nonsuicidal youths and that continued youthful suicidal behavior may be associated with an inability to achieve adequate family relationships. Loss of a parent, family conflict, and a variety of dysfunctional parental characteristics such as emotional problems, health problems, and negative attitudes in parent-child relationships are contributing factors.

Others have found family stress, especially that resulting from marital and parent-child conflict, to be a key factor in suicidal tendencies in adolescents. According to Joseph Sabbatch (1969, 1971), adolescents attempting suicide tend to see family conflicts as longstanding and extreme. They describe their homes as filled with frequent quarreling, distress, and emotional disorganization; there is acute resentment of parents and/or stepparents, accompanied by decreasing communication. Indeed, serious conflict between the adolescent and the parental figures has been described as the single most common event triggering adolescent emergency referrals associated with suicide attempts or threats (Mattsson, Seese, and Hawkins 1969).

Even in cases where the principal problems are in the larger context, the family mirrors and often exacerbates the external pressures felt by the adolescent. An unstable family can make it more difficult for the adolescent to handle outside stress, causing it to seem even more catastrophic than it is. As the essential agent for buffering the pressures of peers, school, and society and for potentially ameliorating suffering, the family is the mechanism through which one's fundamental sense of self and well-being are maintained. Thus the context offered by the family must be made as supportive and coherent as possible.

A lack of coherence in the family context can produce the uncontrollable contradiction and despair that characterize the depressed adolescent in transition to suicide. In order to resolve the acute and profound self-contradictions that undermine the adolescent's self-esteem the therapist must find the paradoxes in the adolescent's context and confront them. It is the therapist's responsibility to work with the system to produce congruence.

In their 1956 article on schizophrenia Gregory Bateson, Don Jackson, Jay Haley, and John Weakland relate the tale of the Zen master's attempt to bring about enlightenment. The master holds a stick over the pupil's head and says, "If you say the stick is real, I will strike you. If you say the stick is not real, I will strike you. If you don't say anything, I will strike you." The schizophrenic, like the Zen pupil, finds himself continually in a situation of paradox, but rather than enlightenment he achieves only disorientation. Similarly, the suicidal adolescent, living in a paradoxical context, only experiences more disorientation when seeking help and confirmation. The essential premises of self are undermined, and it is this disorientation, from which there is no exit, that leads to the suicidal despair in which the only recourse is dissolution of self.

COMMON FAMILY PATTERNS

Triangulation

In the families of suicidal adolescents, there are a number of possible patterns and paradoxical situations that engulf the adolescent. One of the most common is triangulation, in which there are fundamental contradictions in the directives to the child. Often these contradictory directives emanate from a split between the parental figures. The home life is marked by divided loyalties, forcing the child to side with one or the other parent and producing enormous stress for the adolescent. The child is constantly placed in a position of alienating one parent while being exploited by the other. Such patterns of chronic triangulation erode the adolescent's self-esteem because of the guilt of hurting one or the other parent. This can create a situation in which the parents' hopelessness is absorbed by the child. Of course, the adolescent can also experience triangulation in the larger social context, being pulled by the demands of peers, school, or other significant forces.

Triangulation undermines the child's sense of security. The message constantly communicated is that the world is not a safe place. In functional family contexts there are subtle ways in which the adolescent learns to handle rejection, so that when it occurs in the outside context it is not devastating. If the adolescent lives in a family where there is constant triangulation and thus constant rejection and guilt, rejection within the larger social context becomes unbearably threatening. There is no safe and supportive home to return to.

The physical changes, the emotionality, the strivings for identity, the sensitivity of adolescents to the vagaries of peer emotions—all these heighten the adolescent's vulnerability to triangulation. The system is undermining an already shaky self.

The Prematurely Disengaged System

One definition of paradox is a self-contradictory statement that at first seems true. For example, an adolescent sometimes seems to be very much like an adult, at least in physical appearance and maturity. We assume, then, that like an adult, the adolescent should be urged and even forced to be autonomous. However, for many adolescents in our culture this situation is paradoxical. Behind the facade of physical maturity is a child who still requires a great deal of guidance, supervision, and nurturance. And often when autonomy is assumed and encouraged a prematurely disengaged system leads to severe depression and suicidal behavior. We must remember that for the adolescent any urgently felt dependency needs are apt to be interpreted as signs of weakness and thus contribute to lowered self-esteem.

As a rule family therapists tend to see more enmeshed than disengaged families, but when a life-threatening problem such as suicidal behavior becomes evident, even the disengaged will come for therapy. In these families premature disengagement has often occurred because the emotional age of the adolescent has been misjudged. The child feels not freed but ejected!

This ejection is a very dangerous situation since, as Emile Durkheim (1951) points out, the greater the density of the family, the greater the immunity of individuals to suicide. These disorganized family situations breed the feelings of confusion, inadequacy, and low self-esteem related to suicidal behavior. When the ejected adolescent finds the external social context difficult to manage, the child does not go back to the family, which is already a place of devaluation and rejection. Dependent on the reflected appraisal of the peer group or other outside forces and lacking family support, the adolescent becomes extremely vulnerable and may turn aggression against him- or herself. The therapist must determine why the family has prematurely disengaged and is no longer available to the child. Very likely the system is in such disarray that it is no longer attuned to the adolescent's needs.

The Perfect Family

Generically, all of the family systems of suicidal adolescents could be described as overly rigid. These systems do not change shape to accommodate to the new developmental demands of family members. A clear example of rigid systems are families that stress perfection. An imperfect self cannot be tolerated in a system that keeps repeating the message, "You have to be happy, you have to be competent all the time." Such systems are extremely oppressive and create a tremendously high threshold for change. The suicidal symptom of the adolescent can be seen as a desperate attempt to produce change.

In treating "perfect" families the clinician must evaluate the family to see whether it is possible for it to confirm the adolescent as a person. The preparedness of the family to meet this need can be tested by asking these questions: (1) When rejected at the peer level, can the adolescent return home to somebody who is mindful and caring? (2) Can the family present a context that acknowledges the self of the adolescent per se, and not just as an achiever? (3) Can the family allow the adolescent self-definition independent of external standards? If the answers to these questions are positive, the family has a cushion of flexibility and will be adaptive to necessary change.

General Principles

CHANGING BOTH STRUCTURE AND AFFECTIVE COMMUNICATION

Therapy with families of suicidal adolescents must do more than ameliorate the dysfunctions of the system. The therapist should be concerned not only with organizational features of structure but also with what flows from that structure—empathy, warmth, and effective communication. After the organizational features are corrected, *then* the therapy should be directed toward helping the suicidal adolescent feel valued and forgiven—toward giving the child not only toleration but a voice.

MODULATING THE IMPULSIVE SYSTEM

In families with suicidal adolescents the message that is constantly reinforced is that the impulsive solution is expected, if not rewarded. One is not expected to wait out anything, certainly not suffering. We can speculate that much of the adolescent's yielding to suicidal impulses derives from this culture of immediate indulgence, a refusal to postpone, an inability to tolerate contradiction or pain.

The family must be challenged if they accommodate to the adolescent's every whim. If every desire is satisfied immediately, the adolescent has no preparation for tolerating the inevitable frustrations of life. The therapist should examine the family context to ascertain whether it is creating so much stress that modulation is virtually impossible. For example, is one parent drinking heavily? Are there individuals who are overly intrusive? Is there a confluence of forces such as poverty or illness?

HELPING THE FAMILY AVOID CREATING A VULNERABLE CHILD

After a suicide attempt there are times when the family becomes overly protective of the adolescent. The family shields the adolescent from normal stresses and challenges and the resulting overprotection impedes development. This can lead to the creation of a vulnerable child. This presents a paradox for the parents: how can they treat their child like a normal adolescent when the child has done something so terrifying? As a result, the parents cannot begin to approach their child in any kind of normal way. This situation is exacerbated when it occurs in a system marked by conflict avoidance, which is often the case.

In these situations the therapist must work to modulate the guilt felt by the parents. If the family persists in seeing the suicidal adolescent as vulnerable and fragile, then none of the key issues will be addressed. The parents will overprotect and not challenge the child, thereby reinforcing the very difficulties that helped create the problem in the first place. Modulating the guilt is one way to prevent continued confusion and suffering. This process involves working toward reorganizing the system and reopening communication. For the therapist's purposes it does not matter whether we are dealing with what appears to be a suicidal gesture or a serious attempt. Both must be seen as danger signals; both demand focusing on the existential significance of the event to generate intensity and open the system to exploration. Indeed, what is necessary at this point is a sophisticated analysis of the communication that occurred around the event, with a therapeutic emphasis on the structuring of alternatives.

Unfortunately—and contrary to family therapy lore—in my experience not all parental systems are emotionally available and willing to work toward structuring alternatives. For example, I recently saw a family in which after a month of intensive inpatient work the parents continued to cruelly berate their suicidal sixteen-year-old son. The psychotic father said repeatedly, "You're stupid, you will never be the man I am. In fact, I can't believe that you will be anything." He said this while the mother was waiting her turn to be just as cruel. (The father, who claimed he had graduated from college at age seventeen, had not been able to hold a job for years. The family was living permanently in a motel while waiting for an insurance claim to be settled.) After struggling to change this system we recommended foster care for the boy.

In an unresponsive system the therapist cannot allow the suicidal youngster to continue to be devalued by parents who do not understand the situation, who minimize the suicidal behavior, or who react by treating the child as a dangerous freak. The suicide attempt must not be allowed to become a barrier, within either the family or the surrounding context, that prohibits the adolescent from getting back into the mainstream. It is the therapist's job to connect with the child and to other outside resources that can be useful and relied upon.

LOOKING AT THE LARGER CONTEXT

We should also keep in mind that it is possible to *over*estimate the family's participation. Many families of suicidal adolescents enter into therapy thinking that they alone are responsible, ignoring the fact that the adolescent lives in a broader context that can be extremely influential. These families act as if they are indeed totally responsible for the life of the adolescent. This belief, of course, denies a fundamental fact of human existence—that people are free and responsible for their actions. Adolescents, for example, may join in suicide pacts or be heavily involved in the drug culture, factors that may play a great part in precipitating the suicidal behavior. The family's automatic assumption of its responsibility, then, can present a distortion for the family therapist.

The common idea that the child's context is provided solely by the parents and that therefore the family *must* have been doing something that provoked the suicidal behavior should be resisted. Such guilt-inducing assumptions help neither the parents nor the therapy. Indeed, these are families where much of the therapist's work involves saying, "You really didn't have such total control of your adolescent's life." Blaming the family for the suicidal behavior often does nothing but freeze the situation. It creates rigidity and fear which only make the family less willing to work on the problems they may have.

BEING AVAILABLE AS A LIFELINE

A good therapist does not always work strictly through the system. In some situations the therapist must be available to act as a lifeline of positive valuation. In conventional family therapy this might imply that the therapist needs to substitute for and displace the family. And in some cases such action is indeed valid, for the family situation is so bad that the therapist as a lifeline is all that keeps the troubled adolescent afloat. There may not be time to bring the family around, and the therapist must act quickly. Hopefully, in time the therapist's valuation of the child will strike a responsive chord within the family and the therapy will move toward bringing the parents into the process of providing the necessary valuation and support.

TEACHING FINALITY

There is an old Hasidic belief regarding parenting: parents should raise children to give them the sense that in one pocket there is a slip of paper that says "for my sake, and my sake alone, the world was created" and in the other pocket is a slip of paper that says "I am but a grain of sand." There are families that do not confirm their children as individuals but do a good job of helping them to understand the limits and finality of things, to see that they cannot completely prevail in the world. Yet it is a commonplace lesson that needs to be taught. We cannot simply wish things to be. In families with suicidal adolescents that fundamental lesson somehow did not get learned, and the adolescent is left with an insufficient appreciation for the terminable and final nature of things. Unfortunately, this lack of understanding can produce fatal miscalculations.

One of the central concepts of the therapy in this book is the notion of developmental estrangement, the idea that the adolescent must come to an introspective realization of a separate self and of a responsibility for that self. Thus it is a key task of the therapy to facilitate the experience of coming to terms with this existential reality of aloneness, mortality, and vulnerability. In the struggle to have and accept this experience, the parents can give encouragement and empathy, but they must not intervene to rescue the child. The emphasis of the therapy is on the respect for the adolescent's need to struggle and overcome challenge with help.

Having considered the lessons of finality and estrangement the therapist must look at whether the family has allowed the youngster to differentiate sufficiently. Problems of overprotectiveness and differentiation can help create a depressive state and can make the adolescent feel more devalued and despondent. However, to work with differentiation early on may make the child feel even more bereft and thus only exacerbate the depression. Addressing such problems should be attempted only after the adolescent has shed the profound depression that makes the situation so vulnerable and dangerous.

Clinical Example:
Faith, Child of Four Warring Parents

Faith, thirteen years old and in the eighth grade, was admitted to the hospital for treatment after an initial suicide attempt. She had taken sleeping pills and antihistamines before going to school, and when she began acting in an intoxicated manner she was referred to the hospital emergency room. The apparent precipitant for the suicide attempt was one of a series of disputes between Faith, her mother, and her stepfather. In addition, Faith had been extremely upset by the continuing overt animosity between her mother and biological father. According to Faith, whenever she expressed warm feelings for her father, her mother became angry.

ASSESSMENT USING THE FOUR-DIMENSIONAL MODEL

History

Faith's parents were separated when Faith was a baby and were divorced a year later. Both remarried. Her mother, a former alcoholic, was a full-time management trainee in a big department store. Her present husband, a refrigeration specialist, was twenty-five years older than she. This stepfather had three grown children but had been in contact with only one of them since his bitter divorce from his first wife. Faith's father and his second wife owned a small gift shop and had a three-year-old son. Faith lived in Virginia with her mother and stepfather and visited her father and stepmother every other weekend. The biological parents had minimal communication regarding Faith, and when forced to talk on the telephone, one inevitably hung up on the other.

Further complications in this system involved the grandparents. The paternal grandparents were a powerful force in the family, with the father remaining very close to his mother. Faith was even more strongly affected by her maternal grandparents, who up till then had had a tumultuous marriage. The maternal grandfather had in the past threatened to kill his son-in-law. At one time this grandfather had also attempted to molest Faith, an attempt that was fortuitously interrupted by a cousin. Apparently the man had a reputation for dangerous behavior, and there are indications that he may have been sexually involved with Faith's mother.

Structure

Faith was triangulated, caught in the middle between her warring parents. The mother was struggling to diminish the extreme closeness between herself and her daughter, while the father was involved with Faith in an unreliable manner. The overall conflict within the system was exacerbated by the conflict between the maternal grandparents. To this already conflict-laden situation must be added the stepfather's estrangement from his former wife and two of his three grown sons. These layers of generational and relational conflict were a heavy burden for this thirteen-year-old.

Development

The obvious developmental pressure was Faith's emerging adolescence. Many of the concerns surrounding her development were those that every family deals with. Because of the conflict between the families, however, the parents' effectiveness in this time of need was greatly diminished. The mother was overinvolved and felt defensive in the face of the father's criticisms. The stepfather seemed compelled to rectify the mistakes he had made with his own children, and as a result he too was overinvolved with Faith, but with much more conflict than the mother had. The father disparaged both the mother's and the stepfather's attempts at establishing a hierarchy; he insisted that he wanted only to be Faith's friend.

Other developmental issues involved the mother and the maternal grandmother. The mother was training at a business some miles away from home, and the traveling only compounded the expected pressures on her as a thirty-two-year-old management trainee with a family. The maternal grandmother was apparently having her own marital difficulties, struggling to decide whether to continue in a destructive marriage.

Process

The central process issue was the tremendous hostility between the families. The paradox for Faith was that she was living the role of a wishbone, pulled in opposite directions by people she loved. In this position Faith naturally felt that if she loved one side, she was betraying the other.

At the same time, Faith was functioning to keep the two sides at odds. She would often express to her father her unhappiness with her mother and stepfather, eliciting his indignation and animosity, of course, even though he was bent on keeping his distance. There was no conflict avoidance as in some other families discussed in this book. These two families had no difficulty expressing conflict. The pattern, however, was that the conflict led only to emotional explosion, not resolution. An available third person would activate to diffuse the conflict, thus returning the system to its paralyzed state.

THE HOMEOSTATIC MAINTAINER

Who was acting to maintain the dysfunctional homeostasis that provoked Faith's suicidal behavior? The father was the most consistent but others assumed the role as well. During therapy, whenever a meeting of the minds appeared to be imminent, one or the other of the parents would act to return things to the status quo. The one person who consistently acted as a co-therapist during the session was the father's wife. Unlike the other family members, this woman seemed committed to resolving old problems and establishing a new, more functional status.

In addition to family members there was another suspected homeostatic maintainer in the system: the mother and stepfather's therapist. This man encouraged the couple to maintain a total boundary between their family and that of the father. Furthermore, the therapist advised them not to tell the father anything about Faith, even positive things, and suggested that there be no coordinated planning for Faith. He thus actively facilitated the unfortunate wall-building between the two families.

THE THERAPY

Often the suicidal adolescent gives signals of depression that are homeostatically handled in such a way that they are denied, suppressed, and deprived of their significance. As a result the system does not correct the systemic problem to provide new balance for the child. So much of the work in family therapy is to amplify the preventive import of the suicide attempt and to exacerbate the homeostatic patterns that need to be shifted. Often, the suicide attempt is on some level intended to break through these patterns and force the parents to reconnect with the child to whom they have not been responding. In some cases this change does not occur.

The task of the therapist is to transform the family system's message to the adolescent so that the message recognizes the worth and competence of the child's self. If, however, the therapist explores the capabilities of the system and finds it inadequate, then the clinician must take on the family's responsibility of providing positive confirmation.

In these extreme cases, the child cannot remain in a system that intensifies a sacrificing of integrity. The therapist must help arrange a new exit, other than suicide, one that allows the self to balance reality—one that allows the adolescent to see that life itself is not miserable and that this is only a particular, difficult time that is subject to change.

The goals in the therapy with Faith and her family were straightforward. Of primary importance was the necessity to begin a new family organization in which all four parents worked as a unit, thus releasing Faith from her tormenting situation. An additional goal was to provide a lifeline for Faith, making it clear to her that there were adults outside the family system on whom she could rely for help.

Yet another goal was to address the extremely dysfunctional relationships with the grandparents, particularly the maternal grandfather, who was potentially homicidal, had attempted to violate Faith, and had a possible history of sexual abuse of other family members. Lastly, the therapy was directed toward helping to create a context of negotiation between and within both families. Given the dissonance that existed, the current system was extraordinarily inflexible. Therefore, it was necessary to have sessions with both families in which a paradigm for effective negotiation was created and modeled.

The first session with Faith and the two sets of parents was held at a metropolitan hospital; the setting only added to the extreme tension between the two families. The therapist for the family, to whom I was consulting, sat next to me. Faith, a tall, gangly adolescent with black hair and deep blue eyes, was in the middle. Bob, the biological father, sat tall and fair next to Helen, his wife, who was instead dark and notably overweight. Opposite them sat Susan, the biological mother, also very tall and lightly complected, and her husband, Matt, notable because of his extreme thinness and pronounced limp.

DR. FISHMAN   So what do you all think about this?
(to no one in
  particular):

MOTHER:	Well, she's here to get help, and the family session is part of the treatment, is my understanding.
DR. FISHMAN:	Now what is it that has occurred?
MOTHER:	I think Faith should answer that. Since she's the one who took the pills, she should say why she did it or . . .
DR. FISHMAN:	Then why don't you ask Faith why she did it.
MOTHER:	Why did you take the pills?
FAITH:	Because I thought you guys were putting me down a lot, and—I don't know—it seemed like you just didn't like me being around and stuff, and I just I didn't like that, so I just thought, well, if it happens, I die, and if it doesn't— I don't know.
STEPFATHER:	By "putting you down" do you mean telling you to do your homework and turn the TV off at 10:30 at night and stuff—is that putting you down?

I was trying to ascertain what kind of family this was. Faith's statement suggested that her serious suicide attempt was in response to a message from the family system telling her that her absence from the scene would simplify things. The stepfather's response raised another possibility: that Faith was just a thirteen-year-old girl dealing with the normal issues of rebellion and discipline as she began to increasingly assert herself. There is obviously quite a difference between these two views.

As the session continued Faith and her stepfather engaged in a dialogue about incidents of her shoplifting and cutting school. Faith was sensitive to her stepfather's accusation of her being stupid. After three or four minutes of this, the stepmother reacts.

STEPMOTHER:	Well, the exact incident they're talking about, I don't know the full story or anything, but it sounds like to me as if they're talking about a problem that's stemming from something else. I don't think she's just not trying. I think the reason she's having trouble is the relationship at home. If children don't have confidence in themselves— you can't ask them to do things if they don't have the back-up behind them which is giving them the confidence and support that they need. I think that's what they're missing. They're just looking at the outside of the problem—not doing her schoolwork. They're missing the important thing—whatever she's missed along the line.

(As the stepfather and Faith continue to disagree, the father, looking angry, speaks up.)

FATHER: The thing I understand from this conversation—the child needs confidence. You got to give a child confidence. I think Faith—if they would give her a chance instead of putting her down all the time, you'd see a change. She would apply herself. She's not ignorant, she's a very intelligent person. She has an athletic ability you would not believe. I'm really proud of her.

I was beginning to see how Faith was torn between the two sides of the family—her mother's side and her father's side. In the rest of this session my goal is to challenge the adults regarding this family split, to make them aware that whatever their animosities toward one another they had to help extricate Faith from her precarious position in the middle. My efforts are focused on getting this message across to the parents in order to produce change in both warring camps as quickly as possible. What follows is a transcription of a number of attempts to provoke change in this system.

FIRST ATTEMPT

DR. FISHMAN: It seems to me the difficult part is that the adults aren't exactly clear on the way to approach Faith on what's best for Faith. During the course of a month she spends time with everybody and clearly you have differences. What Faith needs so she won't feel so confused and so she won't feel somehow criticized, is that all of you agree.

STEPFATHER: Well let me rephrase my question. (To Faith:) If you're doing the best you can, and you get a C that's okay with me.

FAITH: Then Mom says that if I get a C, I have to take seventh grade over.

MOTHER: When did I say that?

FAITH: This year.

MOTHER: Yes. The first semester we did not question her about what she was doing, other than occasionally ask do you have any homework, what did you do in school. We didn't know how she was doing until after she got her report card. But sometime in January we became aware of the cutting school problem. And it was pointed out to her that you cannot get away with it. So we cracked down on her this semester. (To Faith:) And you know that don't you? We didn't bug you at all last semester, did we? Think about it.

(The mother and stepfather continued to discuss grades with Faith, who responded defensively. The father was visibly angry and moved forward in his chair.)

DR. FISHMAN *(to the father)*:	You're reacting. Why are you reacting?
FATHER:	This is ridiculous. She just told you herself, she cracked down on her. The way I would have solved the situation would be not to crack down on the kid, but to say, "Hey, honey, you've got a problem, let's talk about it. Somebody said you were cutting school. I don't care if you were cutting school, that's between you and yourself—you deal with that. But I want you to come to me and talk to me if you have a problem; let's sit down and work it out." I'm not going to come down on the kid and say you have to do this or else. That's not the way to deal with things.
STEPMOTHER:	I'm just wondering, everything seems to be revolving around the schoolwork. Is that really the problem? If you were doing good in school, would everything be all right? That's what it sounds like, and I just don't think . . .
FAITH:	No. Some of it has to do with home and stuff.
STEPMOTHER:	With what, Faith?
FAITH:	Like the beginning of the year I used to be on the phone a lot, and they got mad at me because of that. But that's stopped now; usually I'm not on the phone. But when I'm supposed to clean the house—and Mom helps too—but I'm supposed to figure out what I'm supposed to clean. *(To her mother:)* And Mom, *I don't know* what you want me to do. You say, "Look around, look what you can do," and stuff. But Mom, I don't know what I am supposed to do.
MOTHER:	So how do you figure out what kind of housework to do? It's what you think you are capable of doing, right? The reason you're not on the phone so much any more—maybe cracked down is not the proper word—you can use any word you want to—but the way of cracking down was, "No more hanging on the phone constantly."
DR. FISHMAN:	You're saying that because your daughter wasn't doing her schoolwork, you said she shouldn't be on the phone.
MOTHER:	Yes, she was being limited.
DR. FISHMAN:	That does make some sense.

> *By supporting the mother I am attempting to get things moving, assuming that the differential support of one member will bring a reaction from another.*

MOTHER: That's what was happening. And it hurt, I know it hurt. There are no other children in the family, so I know her friends are important.

(The father is now visibly agitated and he responds, in turn causing the stepfather to intervene.)

FATHER: Oh, boy. (*To the mother:*) It's your attitude. You've got an attitude problem. You don't know how to deal with kids. When I was married to you, you didn't know how to deal with her.

STEPFATHER (*to the father*): You didn't care whether she starved to death or not.

(Both wives turn toward their respective husbands with calming motions.)

FATHER: Wait a minute, I want to hear this; you want to bring up some dirt, we'll bring up some dirt.

STEPFATHER: That's why we're here I thought.

SECOND ATTEMPT

DR. FISHMAN: No. We're not here for that. We're here for one very simple reason. This girl has four parents. If you parents can bury some hatchets, she won't be doing things like this— she won't have to. If you can't bury hatchets and speak to her with one voice, if you can't agree on what all four of you are doing, she is going to grow up very confused. She is in a very dangerous position. Whatever has happened is water over the dam. Everybody is equally at fault, even though nobody believes it. The only reason we're spending our time here—we're not doing marriage therapy, or divorce therapy or anything like that—the only reason is for Faith. Is everyone agreed that that's why we're here?

STEPFATHER: To help Faith, that's why I'm here.

FATHER: Of course, we're here to help Faith.

DR. FISHMAN: The way to help Faith—it's not easy, but it's very simple. All four adults must be clear on what they want from her and what the consequences are.

FATHER:	There's only one thing wrong in this whole session here. We're here to help Faith, but if her mother doesn't get help, there's no sense in her getting help.
STEPFATHER (*pointing at the father*):	Have you gone to your analyst yet?
MOTHER (*to the stepfather*):	Please, honey.
DR. FISHMAN:	Maybe you're not ready. Maybe you're not ready for us to start.

(*Faith is sitting with her head down and her eyes closed.*)

FATHER:	I asked them to get her a psychiatrist and they wasted ten days. This is why she's in here. I wouldn't have wasted ten days.
DR. FISHMAN:	If you're going to call each other names and cast aspersions we're going to get noplace.
STEPFATHER:	All I'm doing is replying. I'm not starting anything.
STEPMOTHER:	Can I say something here, please? This business about us all getting together. We have tried—and I don't know how to say this without your saying that I'm blaming somebody—but over the years we have not been included in Faith's life. Up until maybe a few years ago, he couldn't even get to see Faith.
THERAPIST:	But we want to start with today. . . .

(*As the bickering among the four adults continues, Faith sits very quietly with her hand partially covering her face and tears on her cheeks.*)

THIRD ATTEMPT

DR. FISHMAN:	The reason for this meeting is because she did something and she could have died.

In order to increase the intensity of the session I reiterate the fact that Faith has made a serious suicide attempt. It is now very important for the parents to emphasize to Faith the notion of finality, since in all probability the girl has no idea of the true significance of her action. By ignoring

*the severity of her act the family implicitly acquiesces in
her denial of her own mortality. If the family can be
brought to show their anguish and upset it would put
Faith's attempt into a clearer perspective.*

FATHER: Faith came to me two weeks ago and told me this isn't the
first time she's done this.

DR. FISHMAN: That makes it even more urgent.

FATHER (*to
Faith*):   What did you say, something like four or five times?

MOTHER: Faith, what did you want out of this session?

*The mother's attempt to stabilize things by including Faith
demonstrates the same triangulation process that led to
the girl's depression.*

(*The intensity has started to build. Faith's hand now covers her face and she is
sobbing softly.*)

DR. FISHMAN: I don't think Faith should stay. I think she should go back
to the room. This really doesn't involve Faith.

*As I see how very sad she appears, I realized that by
keeping Faith in the room we are only emphasizing for
her the seeming hopelessness of the two sides of her
family ever getting together.*

MOTHER: I do think Faith wants to say something about what she
wanted out of this session.

DR. FISHMAN: That's not her job. It's our job, and your job—the adults.
And from all our experience as family therapists, we know
that Faith needs to live in a world where all the adults
agree on what is best for her. What's gone before is water
under the bridge.

THERAPIST (*to
the mother*):   Do you agree that Faith should leave?

MOTHER: Yes, yes.

(*Faith leaves the room with the therapist, who returns a few minutes later.*)

FOURTH ATTEMPT

DR. FISHMAN: I can tell you on the basis of experience and the basis of research, if your daughter is not to do things like she has done, if she is to grow up so that she is not conflicted, the four of you have to speak to her with one voice. Here's what I would suggest. Let's bring up specific issues that need to be addressed—areas where you disagree—and resolve them so that you can agree on what's best for Faith.

STEPMOTHER: One thing, since she really lives with them, and only visits with us, it's very hard for us to know what they're going through. The homework, the cutting school—we weren't aware of that. There have only been a couple of times she's brought her homework along.

DR. FISHMAN (*to the mother*): Do you need more support from this family, from father and stepmother?

MOTHER: Faith comes home and she doesn't talk about their family over here. And she is not to talk about our family when she's over there. That is what I've asked her, because I do not wish to know what is going on over there. And that was the idea of the counseling back in March. She spoke to the counselor, and she came out and said, "I can handle it myself."

STEPFATHER: You asked about *more* support. I don't think we have *any*. We're going to have to go back a bit here, a year or two. (*To the father and stepmother:*) I spoke to you on the phone and you said you're always there to pick up Faith when you say you'll be there. And you're talking to a guy that sat for half, three-quarters of an hour waiting for you to pick her up, because you overslept. And this is a regular occurrence. So I used to take her with me, which upset you.

MOTHER: Yes, but that was solved, Hon, by . . .

STEPFATHER: Yes, lately you've been on time.

DR. FISHMAN: So that's what you want? You want it so you can depend on each other?

STEPMOTHER: But lately it hasn't been like that. I think that's what you're saying. It was a problem a while ago, but it's not really the problem right now. Right?

STEPFATHER: Right. But if I had not treated it the way I did it would be a problem.

DR. FISHMAN: Are there other areas that need support—for example, the music and the schoolwork?

STEPFATHER: I would love it if she would take her guitar over there and practice. She does not practice it enough. She enjoys playing it when she feels like playing it. And I would never say she's stupid. But she will not do her homework unless she's forced to. Like we were discussing—I would come home and there she'd be on the telephone for over an hour.

DR. FISHMAN: So where would you want support? On the guitar? On the cutting school? On things like that?

STEPFATHER: Yes. I don't think it should be necessary to tell the child four times before she'll do it once. This should not be necessary.

STEPMOTHER: We were never told about the cutting school. They never did come to us and say, "Could you help us," or "Could she bring the guitar?" So, it's all right with us if she brings the guitar. We'd be glad to help if she'd bring it over. If there's a cutting school problem—no one ever has asked us to help. That's what I was saying about being left out.

DR. FISHMAN: You would like to be included more.

STEPMOTHER: Yes.

FATHER: Oh yes. (*To mother:*) It's been more than ten years since we've been divorced, and how many times have I been included in something? How many times have you called me up and said, "She has a gym meet in school, would you want to come?" or things like this?

> The father here is speaking to the chronicity of the situation—more than ten years of lack of coordination, more than ten years during which Faith has been shuttled between two very separate homes, with each parent approaching her from a different direction.

The stepmother's reaching out signaled an opportunity to begin some bridge-building. I decided it might be too threatening to introduce the prospect of direct communication among these people and that it would be more useful to present myself as a neutral third party through whom they could begin to open channels of communication.

DR. FISHMAN: So you would like that?

FATHER: Yes. There's no communication here, for one thing.

DR. FISHMAN (to the mother): What about that? You don't necessarily have to talk to each other, you can talk to us.

MOTHER: I said earlier, what works best for Faith and I, is that what goes on in our house we solve at our house, and their problems, they solve at theirs. Now, Faith would like what you're saying—our all working together. But when it comes down to doing it, I called him (*indicating the father*) the day Faith took the overdose. That very day he told his mother that I didn't call him, that Faith called him from the hospital.

This is new information. Clearly, Faith and her mother have talked about the split in the family and Faith has communicated her desire that the two families come together, but her mother has apparently told her that that would be impossible. Could Faith's suicide attempt have been an effort, conscious or unconscious, to create sufficient crisis to fulfill her wish?

FATHER: I don't know where you get your information.

STEPFATHER: From your mother.

FATHER: Well, my mother is a very confused woman.

MOTHER: I do not care to ever call over there, and haven't for a long time, unless I absolutely have to.

A new problem has been introduced: the involvement of the grandparents. The father had a very close relationship (perhaps too close) with his mother, who for many years bailed him out whenever he acted irresponsibly. Somehow the grandmother was involved in the communication difficulties on the occasion of Faith's hospitalization.

DR. FISHMAN: How about things like a gym meet? Things like that—would you be willing to have this family involved? To have her father be involved?

> *I direct my efforts toward bringing the group down to a more mundane, less emotionally charged level.*

MOTHER: I don't know. I have no idea at this point.
STEPFATHER: Something like that, I would prefer if Faith would have a voice in it also.

> *The stepfather assumes the role of the homeostatic maintainer.*

DR. FISHMAN: Assuming that she wants it.

I acquiesced to Faith's having a voice only to keep the dialogue moving. In this system, where the dysfunction is created by the repeated introduction of triangles, including Faith in the decision-making process would only serve to render the system more inefficient and to continue the triangulation. The stepfather's desire to bring in Faith was an attempt to undermine attempts at negotiation. It is clear that the people in the room cannot successfully negotiate the issue if the final decision rests with Faith, who not only is not present but is in no position to arbitrate her own precarious situation within this divided family system.

MOTHER (*to the father*):   Faith would have been very hurt if we told you about what's going on. About what she should have done or she shouldn't. Because she still feels that she has to be very good at your house.
STEPMOTHER: Why does she feel that?
MOTHER: Because Daddy won't see her any more if she's not very good.

> *Here another possible component in the suicidal drama is raised. Faith apparently feels that she has to be perfect for her father. It is possible that in this inflexible system the child has experienced so much past rejection that she fears one more transgression will cause her father to desert her completely.*

(*Both father and stepmother groan and shake their heads as if completely disgusted.*)

FATHER: Oh—we're going down dusty roads here.
MOTHER (*addressing Dr. Fishman*):   All I can say is, before things can move on, that has to be talked out with Faith.

DR. FISHMAN: I hear what you're saying, and I think it's important. But the issue is between Faith and her father. We can help with that in a separate session.

MOTHER: But because of the way Faith feels, it would hurt her more to know that her dad knows. You see? Do you understand that? Because she feels she's got to be good!

STEPMOTHER: Where does she get the idea that she has to be good. That doesn't make sense.

DR. FISHMAN: What we're doing is, we're putting together a series of different sessions. That's a different session. (*To the mother and stepfather:*) That doesn't involve you. That's between Faith and this set of parents (*indicating the father and stepmother*).

FIFTH ATTEMPT

DR. FISHMAN: One way of looking at what Faith did is that Faith is attempting to change things here, among the adults. There's a lot of pain, and I would imagine that, as in every family, everybody is equally right and equally wrong. The point is to work together so that this girl can go through her adolescence. You have a challenge before you so that she can grow up in a way that is not troubled.

MOTHER: Faith and I have already talked about that. What she's wanted . . .

FATHER: What you wanted, not what she wanted.

MOTHER: It's what she wanted.

FATHER: And a while ago it was "what Faith *and I* want"—and really she meant "what *I* want." She's been a manipulator all this time. She's been dealing with us and she's been making everything fine for herself—not for us.

DR. FISHMAN: Are we ready to move on?

MOTHER: What we're asking is what Faith wanted.

STEPFATHER (*to Dr. Fishman*): You're asking for a miracle.

I am becoming increasingly pessimistic. Every effort to encourage negotiation seems to be quickly derailed. However, I decide to make another attempt.

SIXTH ATTEMPT

DR. FISHMAN: I don't think you have any choice but to provide a miracle or she'll grow up very very disturbed. It may be a miracle, but it also requires some grown-up behavior.

FATHER: I made a mistake when we got divorced; I should have taken custody of her and you would have never gotten to see her—only under my conditions. And see how you would have reacted. That would have been a test for you. All these years we've been going through hell, and now you want to turn around and make everyone think that you're such an angel. Well, you're not. You and your whole family, your sick father—you know I could bring up some really bad things about him. He threatened me with a knife. He tried to molest my daughter.

STEPFATHER: You tried to molest your little cousin, too, at the family picnic.

FATHER: Who?

DR. FISHMAN: Listen, I don't know whether we're going to get anywhere.

STEPFATHER: I think we might be better off with private sessions. You get their side and our side, and then you try to sort it out.

FATHER (to the stepfather): You better clean up your backyard before you start throwing stones. Because I know more about her than you think I do.

STEPFATHER: I don't have any stones. I've been throwing them back.

FATHER: You're throwing accusations. You show me the proof. I'll show you the proof.

MOTHER: All right. We do know, I do know—Faith and I know what you want. Faith and I did sit down before she went to this counselor in March. I pointed out why I did not think it would work.

DR. FISHMAN: What would work?

MOTHER: Why it would not work that we could get these two sets of parents making these decisions together. Because as I said, I won't call over there unless I absolutely have to because we always end up in arguments. Now from Dad's [the grandfather's] side—that answer you'll have to get from Faith.

STEPMOTHER: Can I say something? Earlier when we said about what they do at their house is left there, and they don't care about what we do—that's a definite difference from how I feel, and how we feel. I have felt ever since she was little that a little child should be able to talk about whatever they want to under these circumstances. Because when they're little—they are just going to say normal things, like, "I went with my mom to the zoo today." Just to say, "That's nice," and make her feel like it's fine to talk about things like that. But don't ask questions, just let her talk. And I remember her saying when she was younger, "I'm not allowed to talk about you unless it's a problem," and she [the mother] still feels that way, I guess. I thought why can't she mention things? That seemed abnormal not to be able to talk about her life at home.

DR. FISHMAN: You're saying you would like to decrease the separation between the two families.

STEPMOTHER: Yes. I think she [the mother] is separating us by saying I don't want to hear about that. I mean I don't want to hear about every little thing; I wish she could have the freedom to mention the simple everyday things, or even if it's a problem, or even the good things.

DR. FISHMAN: So you think it would be good to bridge the two families. With the good things, not telling each other's business.

STEPFATHER: I have no difficulty with conversations on the phone, it's the two of them (*indicating the father and mother*) that can't talk.

DR. FISHMAN: So you agree with that philosophy?

It is my guess that by moving the emphasis away from the biological parents and making an effort through the stepparents, who are potentially less angry, the system might start changing. I continue on that track, trying to make co-therapists of both stepparents.

STEPFATHER: I have no problem.

DR. FISHMAN: Or if there's a difficulty that needs to be bridged?

STEPMOTHER: Yes.

STEPFATHER: I agree. I've called over there. I'm the one that called up and told you visiting hours and everything, how to get there.

MOTHER: Yes, they [the stepmother and stepfather] can get along all right.

STEPFATHER: But there's an awful lot of animosity between the two of them (*indicating the father and mother*).

DR. FISHMAN: It may well be that it's hopeless, that they can't get over it. There are a lot of marriages where the marriage was a success, but the divorce fails.

FATHER: This is all a farce, you know. I mean this is a part of my life that I'd like to forget. I mean, I was twenty-four when I married her. I must have been a little sick when I did it.

DR. FISHMAN: The fact is, with all due respect—can you forget it?

FATHER: Oh, yeah, it's all over now.

DR. FISHMAN: Tell me one reason why you can't forget it.

STEPMOTHER: Because she's still a reminder.

DR. FISHMAN: Yes. Had you not had children you could have just gone on.

STEPMOTHER: But the child is in the middle, in a sense—although no one ever puts it that way.

DR. FISHMAN: You know something, she loves you just as much as she loves them.

STEPMOTHER: Sure, we know that.

FATHER: And I know she doesn't want to hurt us, and she doesn't want to hurt them. Maybe that's why she gets quiet.

STEPMOTHER: We know she's been in the middle. That's what has always bothered us, but you know—(*to the father*) you have a temper, and just Susan's voice gets you mad. (*To the mother:*) And although you might not lose your temper, you hang up on us.

FATHER: Susan doesn't get so mad, but she hangs up on the phone all the time.

STEPFATHER: He hung up the last time, though.

FATHER: The reason I hung up was she waited until she got home to call me. Something happens to my child, I want to know right away.

The stepmother has begun to provide some perspective to both parents. But when the parents start grumbling at each other again about a past transgression, I decide to intervene.

SEVENTH ATTEMPT

DR. FISHMAN:	The question is how to get this girl out of the middle.
FATHER (*to the stepfather*):	I don't have anything against you, Matt. I think you're an intelligent person. I just can't get along with her (*indicating the mother*).
THERAPIST:	Did you hear Dr. Fishman's question?
FATHER:	No. I wasn't listening.
THERAPIST:	His question was how to get Faith out of the middle.
STEPFATHER:	I've had quite a few quiet talks with her and told her that I don't like her being put in the middle. But I must agree with Susan that what we do at our house, stays at our house. Now if he asks her how she's doing at school, fine. But what we're doing, what we bought, or . . .
STEPMOTHER:	No, no. I mean when it's dealing with Faith herself.
STEPFATHER:	Day-to-day stuff concerning her, neither one of us objects to it. But we had the feeling she was being pumped over there.
STEPMOTHER:	For what?
STEPFATHER:	What we were doing and everything else.
STEPMOTHER:	Only if we thought she was depressed about something, or was having a problem. If we pumped her it was because she wouldn't talk about what was bothering her and she's got to get it out, that's all. Because we only see her on the weekends, and you don't come to us and tell us what's going on. So, we're on the outside, feeling that there's a problem and not knowing where to start.
DR. FISHMAN:	Would you like to be included?
STEPMOTHER:	Sure, that's why we're here.
DR. FISHMAN:	Would you like, for instance, to have Matt [the stepfather] call you and tell you what's going on? So that when she comes over you get a sense of how her life is going?
MOTHER:	You can't do that without talking to Faith first.
DR. FISHMAN:	Of course, but assuming it's all right with Faith.
STEPFATHER:	The answer is yes.
DR. FISHMAN:	Would that be all right with Susan [the mother]?
STEPFATHER:	I think if Faith really wanted it.
DR. FISHMAN:	Ask Susan.
STEPFATHER:	Well, she's not going to be 100 percent, I can tell you that ahead of time.
DR. FISHMAN:	Ask her anyway.

STEPFATHER: Would that be okay—if I called Helen and went over things?

MOTHER: I do not know, because I don't know how Faith feels about it.

STEPMOTHER: Assuming Faith wants it.

STEPFATHER: If Faith would say she would like to have it that way? I certainly have no objection to it. It's not as though we were old friends . . .

DR. FISHMAN: That's not the point.

MOTHER: But see, that is the point. Faith doesn't want it to happen. If we're going to be in the same room and we can't get together—Faith and I did talk about this, we really did.

STEPMOTHER: Talk about what, us getting together?

MOTHER: Yes, we can never be together—we can never be together in the same room.

STEPMOTHER: Well, we're not going to have a family dinner or any-thing—we're talking about Faith.

DR. FISHMAN: We're talking about both parts of Faith's life being there for her.

MOTHER: We can't be together in the same room—that's not going to work.

STEPMOTHER: Like if she's in a gym meet and we're at one end of the auditorium and you're at the other—that's not going to bother her, to know that we're in the same room.

DR. FISHMAN: Assuming that the four of you are grown-up.

An incongruity seems to have surfaced. On the one hand, Faith seems to desperately want both her parents to be together; on the other hand she doesn't want them together in public. As we continue the session it be-comes apparent that Faith is afraid her parents would embarrass her by going to war with one another in public.

STEPMOTHER: Did you ever ask her?

MOTHER: Yes, and she didn't trust it.

DR. FISHMAN: She didn't trust you? She thinks you're childish, that's all.

MOTHER: We'll make fools of ourselves, and it embarrasses her.

DR. FISHMAN: We're making the assumption that you're grown-ups.

STEPFATHER: She's afraid we'll get into an argument in front of her friends and embarrass her.

STEPMOTHER: Well see, that's because this hasn't ever happened be-fore—that we can sit down and talk. This is the closest it's ever come.

DR. FISHMAN:	The question is, can you be decent and distant to each other? We're not going to resolve anything. It's just for the girl, it's only for Faith.
STEPFATHER:	That's why we're here—for Faith.
DR. FISHMAN:	That's why you're all here, why you're all going through this, which I'm sure is very unpleasant.
STEPMOTHER:	But it is going to stay the same if we take the attitude that we can't work it out. Unless we can talk enough to carry it out, to say, "Look, Faith, we're going to try to get along. We both want to see you at the gym meet. So we won't sit together, but we'll be in the same room, and we won't cause a scene, and we won't embarrass you, because we all love you and we're proud of you and we want to make you happy." So if we don't start somewhere . . .
DR. FISHMAN:	Each of you ask your spouses.
STEPMOTHER (*to the father*):	Honey, you'd love to go to gym meets, wouldn't you.
FATHER:	Sure I would.
STEPMOTHER:	Now if we went, and they were there, and we saw them, what would you do? We'd just sort of walk the other way, right?
MOTHER:	Faith doesn't want us walking the other way.
DR. FISHMAN:	Listen, I'll tell you something. It's not Faith's choice. You love her very much, she loves all of you, she shouldn't be caught in the middle at all. The four of you have to decide. When you were thirteen, if you were in the same situation, would you have wanted your parents there—assuming they were grown-up enough to behave themselves? (*To the mother:*) What would you have wanted?

(*The mother leans over and talks quietly to the stepmother.*)

STEPMOTHER:	Can I say something? Susan just said—she said even if we just walk in and walk the other way, she said Faith doesn't want even that, unless we can talk. Now, would that be pushing it? Would that be asking too much? To say, "Look we might not talk, but it's just a start."
DR. FISHMAN:	It's just a start.
STEPMOTHER (*to the mother*):	See, you can say that. At least we're trying. If we get through it and we're all there and we don't have an argument in front of her, that would be one step up.
DR. FISHMAN:	Is each of your spouses willing to do that?

FATHER:	Yes, I'm willing to do that, sure.
DR. FISHMAN:	Matt?
STEPFATHER:	I'm willing to go if she is. I'm sure there's not going to be any conversation, but she's still his daughter.
DR. FISHMAN:	You'd better ask your wife.
MOTHER:	I have one statement. (*To the father:*) Are you going to continue telling Faith to tell her schoolmates that she's a Polack?
FATHER:	Where are we digging this one out of?

Clearly, in this session different people have assumed the mantle of homeostatic maintainer. The four were close to an agreement when the mother brought up the divisive issue of the father's ethnic origin. I had to work to get them back on track to produce closure and to establish the beginnings of a new organization. Eventually even the mother, somewhat reluctantly, agreed that the four adults would decide the gym meet issue, saving Faith from having to decide between her two sets of parents.

A week later there was another joint family session. Just before this session the therapist and I met with Faith alone to learn how things had gone in the previous week and how she was feeling. Had her depression lifted? Was she no longer suicidal? How well was she doing with the other kids on the unit and in the classroom? The answers to these questions would be indicators of how well the parents were doing in creating a new system in which Faith would no longer be triangulated.

DR. FISHMAN:	How about some of these suicidal feelings and actions that you had? Where is that?
FAITH:	Like, yesterday, I felt, why couldn't I have died, and stuff.
DR. FISHMAN:	Why, what upset you?
FAITH:	Things that have happened here—something that happened between this girl and me. So I got mad and stuff, but I got over it.
DR. FISHMAN:	This was a split-second thought? For a few minutes you felt like dying?
FAITH:	Yes, I wished I'd died.
THERAPIST:	Do you feel like you know more alternatives to feeling suicidal?
FAITH:	Yes, I talked to the person and we worked it out.
THERAPIST:	And is that something you've learned here—about talking with people?
FAITH:	Yes, to talk and stuff.

DR. FISHMAN:	So what do you think has changed in your family, or whatever?
FAITH:	Nothing in my family at all. I'm able to communicate more with people.
DR. FISHMAN:	What about your family?
FAITH:	My family? I'm able to communicate with my dad and my stepmother. And Matt talked to me a little bit; we were able to talk. But me and my Mom, we've just not been working things out.
DR. FISHMAN:	Do you see that as kind of a major problem at this point?
FAITH:	Yes. (*She pauses and fidgets, saying nothing.*)
DR. FISHMAN:	How do you see the problems with your parents?
FAITH:	I don't know. You say they ought to be much stricter with me, and I'm sorry, I don't agree with that.
THERAPIST:	Well, we want to know your opinion.
FAITH:	Well, I think they're strict enough. It's one of the reasons why I'm—I don't know. I think it'd just be like, "Do this," and "You can't go out," I don't know.
DR. FISHMAN:	You mean you're not treated like someone your age, you're treated more like a little girl?
FAITH:	Well, they want me to do the work at my age. But then I can't be allowed to go out or anything. Ever since she [the mother] went to school, I've got to help her.
DR. FISHMAN:	In what way?
FAITH:	Well, like I had to do more and more every night. I can understand that because she's not home as much. But— she's always like, "Here, help me with the housework." You know, I've got homework to do, too. At the beginning I didn't do it because I didn't understand that it was graded. So I copied other peoples'. But they won't listen to me when I say that.
DR. FISHMAN:	So being heard is part of your problem?
FAITH:	Yes.
DR. FISHMAN:	How about with your dad and his wife?
FAITH:	It's all right with him. I mean, he understands me and everything. The only thing is—I don't know—he's trying to be with me more when I go over there. But he got mad because I said I was always with Brian [her three-year-old half-brother]. I felt that I was always babysitting and not getting paid for it. And we got in a big argument, and I didn't want to go over there for a while. Stuff like that. But, I mean, we worked things out; we were able to talk to each other.

DR. FISHMAN: So that's better?

FAITH: Yes. It's just—I mean, in a way I'd like to live with them, but I don't want to live with them because, I don't know, I just feel I'd be with Brian the whole time.

DR. FISHMAN: A built-in babysitter?

FAITH: Yes, and I don't want to do that.

Faith clearly was no longer the depressed, waiflike creature of the first interview. She had much more energy, more bounce to both her walk and her voice, and her affect was much more animated. Faith's complaint about her mother seemed the very normal complaint of a thirteen-year-old girl emerging into adolescence who has suddenly had increased household responsibilities foisted on her. We saw it as separate from the pathology of the system.

As the parents entered the room upon Faith's departure, they all seemed more at ease, perhaps because in the past week of therapy they had become more accustomed to being in each other's presence.

DR. FISHMAN: How do you think Faith is doing?

MOTHER: I don't know, I haven't talked to her for a while. I don't think she feels we're working together.

DR. FISHMAN: As a family?

MOTHER: Yes.

DR. FISHMAN: I'll tell you some of our observations about Faith. She seems like a very gentle and a very fine girl.

MOTHER: Yes, she is.

DR. FISHMAN: But also, like every girl her age, she's very fragile. Which we all were, too, at thirteen. Because what she did is very scary. Sometimes kids, even if they're not serious about killing themselves, they have no idea how little it takes.

MOTHER: I think even though she feels that we're not working together, she's still hopeful that we can, she's hopeful.

DR. FISHMAN: I think that all of you did a lot of work. I know how tough it must have been for all of you. There are many hatchets that you have to bury, a lot of difficult times.

The mother seemed to receive the message from Faith and the therapist: "For God's sake, get the parents to grow up and get their act together"—a sign of real progress. My goal at this point was to find out whether she and the rest of the system have indeed changed enough to release Faith from her untenable position in the middle. As the session continued, however, the name calling, casting of aspersions, criticisms, and accusations all revived. The father vehemently denied the accusation of improper behavior toward his niece and offered to take a lie detector test. Needless to say, these goings on made me skeptical that anything had really changed. I therefore decided to proceed by repeating the message from our last session.

DR. FISHMAN: The four of you know the situation, the challenge—and I mean it as a challenge—how can you find a way of working together? That's what Faith needs.

THERAPIST: The area that a week ago you had succeeded in reaching agreement on was the hypothetical gym meet.

STEPFATHER: Well, if Faith wants them to come, fine.

STEPMOTHER: I thought we cleared that up.

MOTHER: It's not up to Faith, remember.

STEPFATHER: You'll be notified, if you want to come, you can come.

FATHER: Can I ask a question? I thought we were here to clear the air.

DR. FISHMAN: I don't think we're really here to clear the air. We can't clear the air. You guys are going to have animosity for the rest of your lives. Are there concrete, specific ways in which you can present a united front to Faith?

STEPMOTHER: I'll just say that we always felt—we always tried to keep Faith out of the middle and tried—we were aware of the two-family situation and so we have tried to keep from saying anything about them. It didn't always work, but we definitely tried and we're going to keep trying. Now, as for what they want to do, how they feel about us—I feel that we can try to keep our personal feelings separate from what we show Faith. And as far as hearing things one way or the other about them, I don't think that's what's important. I feel that at this point what's important is how Faith is feeling.

DR. FISHMAN: I feel the same way about Faith.

The Mother and stepmother clearly have gotten the message. Have the men?

MOTHER: I just feel that these things—things involving Faith and her father are very touchy to me. (*To the father:*) I don't know if you can understand that, Bob. But I would not want to see any child in that position; not just Faith, but any child.

DR. FISHMAN: I think everybody feels the same way. Everybody wants to protect Faith.

FATHER: Faith said some things about you two that I can't believe, but I've never brought that up either. And if you ask me why I'm not bringing them up, it's because I don't have the proof. So I would not have the gall to bring them up to you in the first place. If I even thought that of you, I would never bring it up to Faith.

STEPFATHER: I would like to hear them. Because we're hearing that she does not want to go over there because all she is is a babysitter over there.

The men have not gotten the message. This is more of the old anger.

MOTHER: Maybe that's something for one of the sessions. Why is she lying like this, if this is the case?

STEPFATHER: We're getting one side about over there, and apparently she's going over there and giving them a bad picture of us.

FATHER: She doesn't give a bad picture of you. It's just—at our last session when we were talking and Faith was with us, she said that you told her to kiss your ass. Did you do that?

STEPFATHER: One time.

DR. FISHMAN: You know, Faith is young, but Faith knows how to play both sides against the middle.

This last comment is my attempt to utilize the circularity of the system. Faith is not just a victim—she is also a protagonist in this complex triangle. In fact, now it is Faith who helps keep the fires of dissent burning.

STEPFATHER: That's what she was attempting to do when I told her to kiss my ass. It seems I made an impression, and I'm glad of it.

FATHER: Now let me explain something to you. I'm her father and I've never talked to her like that. You're not her father, and you shouldn't talk to her like that.

STEPFATHER: You have no idea why I said it.

DR. FISHMAN: And that's exactly why—both of you are out of context.

STEPFATHER: Well, my son says "fuck you" to me, and that's the first time he's ever talked like that to me, and I didn't return the thought back to him. I wouldn't have the guts to do that—maybe you're overreacting. You've got to use your head. You're an adult.

DR. FISHMAN: The fact is she's a child, and the fact is she knows how to play you guys off against each other.

STEPFATHER: She tries.

DR. FISHMAN: Well, what do you think is the way out? This is your family. This is the situation you have created.

STEPMOTHER: Well, I've been aware of Faith playing between us, so the few times she said anything about them, I was aware not to let it—I know their feelings, I know they don't like us, so I'm careful not to take sides.

DR. FISHMAN: Are you suggesting something? Are you suggesting that when these things happen, you will call the others? What about that?

Playing up this suggestion is my attempt to create a new organization in the form of a new social convention. There needs to be an open channel, a hotline between the two families, so that when there is upsetting information from Faith, either family can pick up the phone and call the other.

STEPMOTHER: I wasn't thinking about that, really.

DR. FISHMAN: Well, what about that? What about calling her mother and saying, "This is what we've heard, let's check it. We adults have to stick together." That's what we're talking about —this is the battle of the generations.

STEPMOTHER: What I'm saying, and I'm not saying it for Bob necessarily, but when she has said anything, I didn't take what she said at face value. The way she's presenting it could be different from how it really happened. So I try to be unbiased about what she says.

DR. FISHMAN: I understand that. Can you check it out?

STEPMOTHER: Yes, if it's something really important that she's saying and I think it's important to know if it's true or not—yes.

DR. FISHMAN: Good.

THERAPIST: I'm not sure they [the husbands] can. Bob still can't talk to Matt about "kiss my ass." It seems like that's still something that needs to be hashed out.

FATHER: Well, let's put it this way, she's my only daughter. If I hear some man talked to her like that, I put him on his ass. I don't like that. They're my kids, it's a touchy subject. I love them both. What I created, he destroyed.

DR. FISHMAN: This is exactly what we're talking about. How can all of you separate some of your egos and say, "Wait a minute!"

MOTHER: My question is, are you (*indicating the father and stepmother*) seeking custody of Faith?

FATHER: I'm not going to lie to you, we talked about it. I think that if she goes back to the same environment and things don't work out, then I might try for custody. But if things change, if the four of us can get together and talk and have a better environment with my daughter—just so when she comes to my house we don't curse at her and we don't say, "You can't do this" or "You can't do that." Kids are really impressionable. If you tell them they can't then they think, well my father won't let me do that, then I don't like my father.

The father's position is that of the peripheral parent. The most important thing to him is that his child like him. He fears that if he establishes a hierarchy and enforces rules, his daughter will not love him. Interestingly, both the child and the father have the same fear of being deserted by the other.

Clearly, the antidote for this peripheral father-daughter relationship is to get the father to become more involved in a parental capacity and not just serve as a weekend buddy. In the last segment of the session, new information indicated that the father himself might be planning moves in that direction. He had been talking about suing for custody, which would represent a new escalation in the war between the families.

DR. FISHMAN: So if the environment changes?

FATHER: If the environment changes, there's no reason to change anything. But there's got to be a change.

DR. FISHMAN: Are there concrete ways that you can all work together?

FATHER: We've got to get close to Faith, for one thing.

The father is absolutely correct. A more genuine relation-
ship with his daughter would help him become more
sensitive to the stepfather's functioning as a parent.

As the session moved on the parents discussed Faith's desire to call
her stepmother "Mother." The father had said at one point that he did not
feel comfortable with that, but with urging from the others he agreed that
it was an issue between Faith and her stepmother and should be left for
them to decide.

My goal is to have these four parents resolve a conflict which would
signal the emergence of a new pattern. I therefore return to a concrete and
observable issue, the gym meet.

THERAPIST:	So, we have a hypothetical gym meet that we've agreed on. What else?
DR. FISHMAN:	Between you two families.
STEPFATHER:	I guess we could call if she tells us something. But I also realize what you said, she'll play one against the other. Kids have a tendency to do that.
DR. FISHMAN:	I can tell you something about adolescents: they're mercenaries. They're working to get what they can. And you guys, because of the split in the situation, are even more vulnerable.
STEPFATHER:	Okay, when I hear a so-called rumor, I'll consider calling over and ask them whether it actually happened.
FATHER:	I'll tell you, it's really hard for me to say this, but I'm ready to forget everything that ever happened to us and to just start all over and try to burn these bridges and get done with all this argument. I'm tired of it. Let's just try and get along together. And if I hear something about you and I don't believe it, I'll call you up, we'll talk about it.

This is an impressive statement from the father. For over
ten years he has been warring with his ex-wife. To agree
now to put the warfare aside and move on is a significant
change, and all I can do is emphasize its importance to his
fragile daughter.

DR. FISHMAN:	Your daughter is a fragile human being—she needs that.
FATHER:	Yes. Maybe I've neglected her a little . . .

DR. FISHMAN: Don't get into that, you have many years to correct the situation. That's not the function here.

FATHER: It scares me, it really does, I don't know where she's at. It's great, you know, to have somebody say "I love you" or "I care about you, I really want you to be around, I want to listen to what you have to say, I have confidence in you."

DR. FISHMAN:
(to the
mother):   What do you think?

MOTHER: I don't know if I should believe her, but I want to believe her.

THERAPIST: Do you believe in this principle of rumor control?

MOTHER: If I say that, when I hear one more thing—Faith will be going over there again . . .

FATHER: Well, this is our stumbling block here. First of all, there's nothing to that. I don't know where you get these things. It's just a rumor.

I believe mother and father are somewhat disoriented by the newness of their changed positions—thus the non sequiturs.

The discussion moved on to rumors of the father's having indiscreetly tickled a niece and the instability of his marriage, problems that had been blown out of proportion. After discussion and explanation the families were able to come to some closure on these topics.

DR. FISHMAN: The important thing is this kind of communication, coming to some kind of understanding about suspicions and fears.

MOTHER: (to
the father):   But when I call you to check it out, I don't want you getting angry at me for checking it out, okay? Is that understood?

FATHER: What do you mean?

MOTHER: If she comes to me with a rumor, I'm going to call you and I'm going to tell you exactly what she said, and I don't want you to be offended.

FATHER: I'm not going to be offended.

MOTHER: No, the things that we've mentioned, the rumors and . . . and the other—I'm pointing out these major rumors, as they say, and I didn't consider them as rumors.

DR. FISHMAN: Ask Matt to call them.

STEPFATHER: I'll call over, verify whether the rumor is true or not, or what Faith is saying—we'll probably discuss it first.

DR. FISHMAN: You probably should.

FATHER: Well, I hope this all comes out, because this really makes me uneasy.

DR. FISHMAN: Okay, the point is to go beyond it, so the two of you are a bridge to one another and Faith doesn't get caught between you. Okay, shall we bring her in now?

(Faith enters the room.)

DR. FISHMAN: Now, is there anything that any one of the four of you want to say in terms of bridges and things like that?

STEPMOTHER: We're in agreement [that] if there's something at school or
(to Faith): something like that, we can all come and be there to watch you and there's no problem with that. Can you understand that?

FAITH: Yeah.

STEPMOTHER: And we talked about getting together, the four of us, and the one thing that we covered today was that since there has been some problem with rumors—you know, things said about us, each of us—that if something's brought up one would call the other and check it out instead of just believing what was said. Because there's been a conflict there that's gotten in the way of understanding what's going on.

MOTHER: It doesn't mean we're checking up on each other and on you, it's just that . . .

FAITH: I hear what you're saying.

DR. FISHMAN: And about gym meets?

MOTHER: She *(indicating the stepmother)* already said that.

STEPMOTHER: Yes, anything to do with school, or some function that we'd be going to.

FATHER: What about school? How are you doing? How are you making out?

DR. FISHMAN: We'll work on that; that's another session. *(To Faith:)* Do you have any questions of your parents? And by parents, I mean all of them.

Much to my pleasure and the therapist's, Faith then created a challenge. She asked permission to go on leave from the hospital in order to spend some time with a friend (and probably get a chance to see the boyfriend she met while in the hospital). The parents' newfound organization was challenged to see if the four of them could resolve together this very normal problem in adolescent control.

The father, always courting the goodwill of his daughter, was an easy touch; after asking a few questions, he readily agreed. But this was too good an opportunity to ignore. All four needed to agree. I asked, "What have the four of you to say?" The mother, stepfather, and stepmother then questioned Faith closely about where she was going, who would be there, and how she would behave.

Faith then left the room to return to class and the therapist and I excused ourselves, while the two families discussed the pros and cons of Faith's request. As we observed from the monitor, we were extremely impressed by the new organization that seemed to have been established. All four parents participated equally in deciding how to make this parental decision. After about fifteen minutes of discussion they were all agreed and the therapist and I returned, along with Faith, to hear the verdict.

FATHER:	We've all talked it over. We've analyzed everything and we don't think we can let you go. We don't think that you're responsible enough right now. Maybe in a little while, if you buckle down and things go well. And if it's something we know more about.
MOTHER:	We think you're doing fine. We really do, except for some of the difficulties in your schoolwork. Other things we've seen you are doing well.
FATHER:	Is there anything you want to say?
FAITH:	No.
STEPFATHER:	We just feel that without knowing exactly where you're going and what you will be doing—well, it'd be a little bit like just dropping you off at the boardwalk.
FATHER:	I've never really said no to you, Faith. But this is something that really worries me. We all talked it over.
THERAPIST:	The four of you?
FATHER:	Yes, we all talked it over.

(Faith leaves the room. As the therapist and I get up to leave the father crosses the room to the stepfather and shakes his hand, thanking him. Then he goes over to his former wife and puts out his hand to her. She takes his hand and holds it tightly, pulling him toward her.)

MOTHER: I don't hate you, you know.

FATHER: I don't hate you either. I want us to stop fighting. We're going to burn these bridges. That's the way I want it.

MOTHER: I've been afraid of you. It took me a long time to be able to talk to you.

FATHER: It took me a lot of guts just to shake your hand.

Summary

With this scene the system seemed transformed.* The four adults appeared finally to be working together. For the first time in at least ten years the father and the mother appeared to be ready to bury some hatchets.

I noticed, however, that while this touching scene was taking place between the father and mother, the stepmother stood in the doorway with her arms crossed over her breast, staring at them. I saw this as the previous organization raising its head. It was a clear reminder of how difficult it is to transform a very chronic system and that there was much more work to be done. But the therapy seemed to have achieved the goal of all four parents living in a system capable of giving congruent messages to the girl. All of them were now acting as her parents.

The following week both families were again able to come to a consensus on a complex issue around Faith's desire to see her boyfriend. They continued in outpatient therapy after Faith left the hospital. They have sometimes used the therapy sessions to air their complaints about one another, but have rallied when necessary to handle problems. At this writing, all involved are committed to therapy. They see that it is in their mutual best interest for the good of their daughter.

I see this as a very good outcome. We cannot hope to transform problems like this family has suffered in only a few sessions or even a few months. But if the therapist can bring the family to be genuinely engaged in therapy, then there is real hope, even for chronically troubled families.

---

* If this chapter has seemed slow moving, the experience is akin to our experience in the treatment room. What we found necessary was an intensity of repetitions—an erosion of the old, dysfunctional patterns.

8

Disability and the Family: The Search for Competence

> The mirror sees the man as beautiful, the mirror loves the man; another mirror sees the man as frightful and hates him; and it is always the same being who produces the impressions.
>
> —MARQUIS DE SADE

DISABILITY IN ADOLESCENTS may be defined as any condition that potentially impairs functioning. The condition may be chronic, such as retardation, or temporary, such as the compound fracture of the leg. Certain disabled children are at risk of being developmentally and psychologically impaired for the rest of their lives. Yet a close examination of the literature on children at risk demonstrates that only a minority of disabled children and adolescents experience serious difficulties in personality development. In fact, the vast majority who are exposed to various forms of adversity develop normally and enjoy productive lives (Hauser et al. 1985). Our concern here, however, is the small number of children who do have severe difficulties.

One way of approaching this minority is to study the majority of disabled children who seem to handle their adversities well. In doing so we can discover the qualities of disabled children and their families that encourage successful coping. There is a rapidly expanding literature on these successful children who become invulnerable or resistant to the risks of their disabilities. These studies reveal a vast number of causes for resiliency, including high self-esteem, capacity to control environment, social and scholastic competence, maternal warmth, and a balanced family interaction. In a study of diabetic children Maija-Liisa Koski (1969, 1976) identifies the children who coped best as those having come from families with clear, distinct boundaries between members, realistic and cooperative attitudes toward disability treatment, low marital conflict, and stable composition with the presence of two parents or a competent single parent. Other studies have found that the parents of children exhibiting optimal control consistently value independence, self-sufficiency, and open expression of feelings (Anderson et al. 1981). And researchers such as Michael Rutter (1979) and Norman Garmezy (1983) emphasize the ameliorative role of social support systems and community institutions such as schools.

Recently I saw a comedian who asked the audience, "How many thought there was something very wrong with you when you were an adolescent?" Virtually everyone in the audience raised their hands. If this is the experience of normal adolescents, think what it must be like for youngsters who do in fact vary from the norm. The presence of a disability can profoundly affect the major developmental tasks of adolescence, such as separation from the family, the establishment of a separate identity, the acquisition of social competence, and the abandonment of childish narcissism. How the family and the larger social context treat the disabled adolescent profoundly affects how the youngster navigates these developmental passages.

My focus here is to build on this research and uncover principles of treatment that will show us how the disabled adolescent's social context—family, school, medical personnel, and social agencies—can become a resource for healing and growth. I believe these principles are important for disabled individuals and their families generally, but even more so for disabled *adolescents*. In the adolescent the psychological processes are inextricably influenced by on-going physical changes. How the social context and, especially, the family treat the adolescent has a profound affect. The disabled child is more vulnerable during adolescence than at any other period in childhood. For the disabled adolescent the difficult problems are more difficult. Their disabilities may render their bodies or their minds less reliable than those of their peers, thus compounding the experience for the ever self-conscious adolescent.

General Principles

When dealing with families with disabled children, often the therapist can change the system simply by using the technique of *adding information* (a technique described more fully in another work, *Family Therapy Techniques* [Minuchin and Fishman 1981]). Briefly, what this involves is gently nudging the system toward change by providing information on other options or ways of coping.

This technique is not always successful, however, especially if one is dealing with a psychosomatic family. In treating these families the therapist must be attuned to the presence of characteristics such as enmeshment, overprotectiveness, rigidity, triangulation, and diffusion of conflict. Such situations require a therapy of transformation in which intensity and enactment are used to alter the prevailing patterns right there in the therapy room, and a careful follow-up to ensure that the changes have transferred to home and school. The case study presented later in this chapter includes a therapeutic consultation with one such family.

WORKING RAPIDLY TO COUNTER PRESSURES THAT REINFORCE THE DISABILITY

With disabled adolescents the therapist must work rapidly toward assessment and intervention to counter any pressures from the family system to see the adolescent *only* as disabled and thus to constantly reinforce the disability. The immediate therapeutic goals might vary depending on the age of the child. With younger adolescents the family system might be encouraged to help the child negotiate capabilities; with teenagers the issue may be to provide challenge in the absence of a close connection to peer groups or a strenuous effort to connect the youngster with a peer group. With older adolescents the focus might be on preparation for leaving home. Whatever the primary issue, the therapist must work to enhance functioning as much as possible in the face of the systemic forces that act to stress the disability.

TRANSFORMING THE CYCLE OF LIMITED EXPECTATIONS

Many families with disabled children fall into an insidious trap. The family expects diminished functioning of the disabled youngster and therefore does not challenge the adolescent to stretch and grow. The adolescent, accepting the family's views, does not strive and so languishes in the disability. I call this trap the "hall of mirrors" phenomenon (Fishman, Scott, and Betof 1977). When someone is diagnosed as disabled the label can create special relationships with other people that result in lower expectations and diminished skills. The way the individual is treated affects his self-concept. If the image reflects only the limitations of the disability, then the person's self-image and potential are diminished because he sees himself as impaired. His response to these reflections in a "hall of mirrors" serves to substantiate the image. The result is a self-fulfilling prophecy.

In order to disrupt this cycle the therapist must establish a context in which the possibility of competence and challenge replaces the self-fulfilling expectation of diminished capacity. To do so the therapist must first determine the extent to which the limited capacity is a function of being treated as a limited person. Conversely, one must also ask how much the deficit of the individual serves to organize people in the social context to treat him as disabled.

The goal of therapy, then, must be to change the dysfunctional patterns of interaction between individual and context. The therapist must work with family members, school and medical personnel, and social agencies to increase not only the expectations but the actual functioning level of the disabled child. Too often the disability in question is seen as a permanent, immutable state, losing sight of the fact that there is always a margin within which the adolescent can improve. Moreover, if the parents or others surrounding the disabled individual communicate a feeling of fixed or insurmountable limitation, then that feeling will become reality: the development will freeze and the likelihood increases that the adolescent will remain dysfunctionally impaired.

RECOGNIZING HEIGHTENED VULNERABILITY

The therapist must be able to dissect how the family's needs are played out in the process of caring for the handicapped individual. There is always the danger that relatives will find too much meaning and purpose in the role of helper. Family members experiencing periods of heightened vulnerability in their own lives—when their own needs are not being met and their frustrations are exacerbated—sometimes find it essential to maintain the disabled child as a patient. They may even begin to enjoy the caretaker role and become extremely reluctant to allow the child to emerge as someone other than a helpless individual. It is clear that for many of these family members focusing on a disabled child is easier than dealing with their own issues. In these cases developmental stagnation sets in and the process of helping the disabled adolescent overrides all other processes. The needs of the disabled member tend to run the family, and the family becomes paralyzed.

As therapists we can direct family members to work on their own issues and to foster their own autonomy. The family therapist can help parents and others to step back and ask, "Am I getting too much out of helping?" By encouraging such reflection and offering alternative behaviors and scenarios, we work to prevent the development of overprotective, psychologically crippling relationships in the family. Our goal is to help parents better provide the energizing free space in which the disabled adolescent can grow, without allowing themselves to be recruited as overly assiduous helpers.

One step toward reaching this goal is to ask ourselves the question, "When is a family most likely to organize itself around the limitations of the disabled member?" It is my experience that these periods of heightened vulnerability occur at life-stage transition points: a job change, a mid-life crisis, a death in the family, or problems in the marital relationship. Exacerbations of the adolescent's illness can also mobilize the focus and heighten the psychological vulnerability of the family.

The therapist must be sensitive to these transition points that affect the family's vulnerability. Often they can help explain cessation of a disabled adolescent's progress. For example, a clinician may be faced with an adolescent whose illness has a self-limited course but who has given up trying just as recovery was in sight. Too late, it is discovered that the father saved himself from depression surrounding a ruptured relationship with his spouse by actively maintaining his child's disability. In other words, he "married" his child to save himself at a difficult time of transition.

The therapist must also recognize that the amplification or maintenance of the handicapped state is extremely easy for families to fall subject to. In fact, it is so easy because it is the handicapped child's prerogative to try to elicit such a reaction from them. The family must understand when this pull on them is occurring and must be helped as quickly as possible to become adept at avoiding it. The therapist's goal is to help the family foster whatever independence the disabled person and the system are capable of attaining.

SEARCHING FOR COMPETENCE

One of the key principles in dealing with disabled adolescents and their families is searching for areas of the child's mastery and competence. By highlighting these areas the therapist can help challenge the developmental expectations of both parents and child. This issue will be discussed in greater detail later, in the clinical example. But it is essential for the therapy to be structured so that the parents and the child are given an opportunity to see the child as competent. By employing a therapy of experience in the treatment room, an area of true competence can be demonstrated and seized upon. Stressing its significance can be critical in breaking down whatever walls of limitation the family and the adolescent may have constructed.

ORGANIZING A NETWORK OF CARE

A family is not solely a help-giving support system; it can also serve the important function of problem resolution. Effective problem resolution, however, frequently involves distinguishing what is best done within the family and what is best done outside it. It is a misconception that when one is part of a family, other family members can always offer the best support. In fact, sometimes a therapist can be most helpful merely by informing family members when they *cannot* support one another—for example, when support would place unrealistic demands on individuals or would overstress the system. At such times the therapist should lead the family to look for extrafamilial resources and to create a support system without undue pressure on any one individual.

In creating this support system the definition of the family can be enlarged, even to include more than just relatives. Some years ago, for example, I worked with a family that included a mother who was a single parent, a sixteen-year-old asthmatic girl, and her eight-year-old brother, who had a severe neurological disorder. The mother was obviously overwhelmed by the enormity of her responsibilities. Our first step was to work within the nuclear family. I taught the teenager a relaxation technique so that, at the earliest possible perception of chest tightening, she could try to prevent an attack. This could only be done in the context of family work, for we first had to decrease the extreme enmeshment of mother and daughter, who were so close that the girl actually expected her mother to know when her asthmatic attacks would come on. Only when the girl "owned" her body and felt the early tightening could she head off the attacks and exercise her competence and mastery. Concurrent with this family work we created an organized context of outside helpers to take some of the pressure off the overburdened mother. This enlarged family network allowed the mother to realize that she could in fact be a good mother without having to do everything for her children. Indeed, she could become a better mother if she let others help and did more for herself, thereby freeing herself to be more productive and allowing her children to grow in competence and independence.

ADDRESSING THE FALLOUT: HOW ARE THE SIBLINGS?

In families where one of the siblings is disabled the clinician needs to ask how the disability has affected the development of the other children. Frequently these siblings are depressed, unattended children who have to spend too much time taking care of an ill brother or sister. The disabled adolescent may take all of the parents' attention, leaving siblings to deal with feelings of neglect, hostility, or jealousy. Even in cases where the illness is of a limited duration or where the disabled child miraculously recovers, the siblings may still suffer. Though they may hope or expect that their parents will now attend to them in a more balanced way, this does not usually happen. Frequently such problems of neglected siblings cannot be solved strictly through intrafamilial work. The parents are simply over-loaded and can only give so much. The siblings need and must be provided another, outside support system. One oncology unit I know of has insti-tuted sibling groups. These do not replace the parents, who must still be encouraged to deal with and support the siblings, but the groups do offer some relief. The members of the group are able to support one another and share experiences, providing a sense of independence and independent problem solving not contingent on the attention of the parents.

Clinical Example:
Ingrid, A Case of Too Many Helpers

The following consultation occurred in Sweden with a nineteen-year-old girl and her parents. Ingrid had been diagnosed as mentally retarded. She lived at home, unemployed, with no pressure to move on either from her parents or the family's helpers. When I saw the family Ingrid was in a psychiatric hospital because of a suicide attempt. This was her first attempt, although she was described as having been depressed for many years.

ASSESSMENT USING THE FOUR-DIMENSIONAL MODEL

History

Ingrid had the classic history of a disabled adolescent. She had been associated with institutions for essentially her whole life. The "hall of mirrors" phenomenon was very much in evidence. The specific event that precipitated the consultation was extreme depression and desperation about her life and future, brought on by a breakup with a boyfriend, which had led to the attempted suicide.

Development

Both parents were in their early sixties and were clearly engaged in a developmental passage, retirement, in a context of socialism, where retirement is rigidly adhered to. Ingrid was the last of four children; when she left home the parents would enter into a new developmental stage—that of having no child at home, a situation they had not faced for more than twenty years.

Structure

The family's relationships, especially when seen in the developmental context, revealed a situation in which both parents were extremely overinvolved with Ingrid. Their overinvolvement was of a flip-flop nature: one would distance and the other would grab onto the girl, and then they would reverse roles.

The other relationships involved were in some ways due to characteristics of socialized Scandinavian societies. Unlike the United States and other countries, Sweden has an abundance of social services, providing helpers at all levels. In this case there was a woman in her mid-fifties whose job was to help Ingrid's day flow more smoothly. The unintended result was that another barrier to Ingrid's possible autonomy was created. Not only did the family have difficulty creating a context for Ingrid to test her wings, but the social system compounded the problem by providing at least one person, and at times several, whose sole job was to do for this girl all those things she was supposedly incapable of doing on her own.

Process

The observed process was that of a psychosomatic family. Both her parents and the involved social agencies were overprotective of Ingrid. Other specific process parameters demonstrated were triangulation, diffusion of conflict, and rigidity.

I was moved by this warm and vulnerable young woman. She was extremely compelling. As a therapist I felt pulled to be drafted as yet one more helper, one more too-helpful professional to be recruited into the service of this appealing adolescent, taking over for her and making it difficult for her to develop her own competence through trial and error. The very urge to do something for this girl helped me to generate intensity while being wary not to be too helpful. Ingrid had to be her own advocate.

THE HOMEOSTATIC MAINTAINER

In this family the homeostatic maintainer appeared to be both parents, who persisted in seeing their daughter as so impaired that she could not work and live independently. To the extent that they had this view, they protected and supported their child's incapacity. Rather than challenge their daughter to grow and expand her possibilities, they maintained the homeostasis. Also maintaining the dysfunctional homeostasis were the social-service helpers, such as the woman who was assigned solely to Ingrid.

THE THERAPY

In the room are Ingrid, a plain and young looking girl, her middle-age mother and father dressed in work clothes, and the therapist. Unfortunately absent were siblings and Ingrid's professional helper. Since I do not speak Swedish, the therapist acts as translator. As the session begins, however, it becomes apparent that Ingrid understands my English.

DR. FISHMAN: Do you know English?

INGRID: Some . . .

DR. FISHMAN: Where did you learn some English?

INGRID: From the TV.

DR. FISHMAN: So you know English but your parents don't. (*To the parents:*) It's great, she really knows English.

(The mother turns to her husband in absolute disbelief.)

MOTHER: It seems she knows more English than we know—than we are aware of.

THERAPIST: I think I will translate for the parents. Okay?

DR. FISHMAN: What do you want as parents for your daughter?

MOTHER: We're not sure what it is.

DR. FISHMAN *(to Ingrid)*:   Will you tell me what your mother said?

An area has been established in which the girl is competent—in fact, even more competent than her parents. In addition, as the session develops everyone can laugh at my incompetence with Swedish, and Ingrid, in a very nice way, becomes my guide.

FATHER: Well, we don't exactly know what she is capable of doing and we're not aware of what her ideas are.

DR. FISHMAN: Are you, Ingrid, also confused? You don't know how independent you can be?

INGRID: I don't know.

DR. FISHMAN: So everybody is confused, you're confused too.

MOTHER: The only time she worked before was after school. And she never has worked for a long period. Never. One or two weeks.

THERAPIST: As part of the school system, you work for a couple of weeks to see what working is like.

DR. FISHMAN: What kind of work do you like to do? What do you want to do?

INGRID: Flowers. I love flowers.

DR. FISHMAN: What is your favorite flower?

INGRID: Cactus. *(Everyone laughs.)*

I was impressed that this girl who likes flowers would choose cactus as her favorite. I surmise that people who choose cactus as their favorite flower are individuals who have been forced to rely on a very dry and barren emotional environment. They are people who are struggling to learn to live on few supplies, just as a cactus makes do with only a little water. Moreover, they are people who become economic; they know they cannot count much on their environment, so they learn to conserve what they have. One might also conclude that Ingrid was trying to ward off intrusiveness. Perhaps, like the cactus, she maintains a rough, thorny exterior, while on the inside there is real nurturance.

DR. FISHMAN:	You know, some cactus are very very big.
INGRID:	Ya, those are my favorite cactus. They're a little like people. (*laughter*)
DR. FISHMAN:	Do you want to get a job?
INGRID:	Yes.
DR. FISHMAN:	You know English. Do you want a job working with flowers?
INGRID:	Yes.
DR. FISHMAN (*pointing to a plant on the windowsill*):	Can you help that one?

Ingrid laughed because the plant was in very poor shape. The therapist whose office we were in was also the venerated director of the clinic, but he knew nothing about plants. Obviously, Ingrid did have some knowledge of plants. This represented another possible area of competence. The psychiatrist took the plant off the windowsill and held it for the girl's inspection.

> INGRID: It's got small animals [mites].

(*She continued in Swedish to instruct the psychiatrist on what to do with his plant.*)

My work here was centered on searching for discovery of the competent self. This search was organized by my knowledge that both the family and the therapist of this retarded girl had been unsuccessful at connecting with that part of Ingrid's multifaceted self that wanted to grow. All of my interactions, therefore, were focused on reinforcing in the girl that aspect of self that was competent and caretaking and could have ascendancy over the others in the room. This required being alert to the available cues (such as her mother saying, "She knows more English than we know"), then capitalizing on and amplifying such cues. In part I was able to do this by emphasizing both my own newness in the situation and my difficulty with the language, placing myself in the position of a beginner who needed to be instructed in all of the details.

Highlighting for this retarded girl a little corner in which she was competent would open up a new reality for the whole family. However, this was not a therapy in which I could just give the family a new reality and wait for new patterns to emerge. It had to be a therapy of active intervention. When Ingrid instructed the prestigious psychiatrist in how to handle his plant, she set the stage for being treated as an adult. This event, then, became not an isolated interaction but part of a central strategy for change. This kind of therapy is unusual in that it acknowledges the ultimate significance of these small events in reinforcing the positive self, the identity that so far has not been attended to.

Countering Induction with a Fast Assessment

In families of the disabled, especially those with retarded children, the adults tend to organize themselves to confirm the incompetence of the youngster, taking over for these children and patronizing them. For therapy to be effective fast diagnosis and correct intervention is essential. The therapist must quickly counter the induction of the adults by finding instances of the adolescent's mastery and competence in dealing with his environment and resist the tendency to focus only on the limited mental capacities of the young person.

In therapy with Ingrid and her family I quickly established areas of Ingrid's competence, challenging the prevailing notions of the adults in the room and dramatically changing their estimation of her potential. It was no accident that at the end of the session the parents had the sudden thought that perhaps their daughter was ready for an attempt to live on her own. Clearly, this radical change was a result of the fast intervention to counteract the induction of the parents and the presiding therapist.

Before we continue, I must emphasize that an important part of working successfully with retarded adolescents is the avoidance of traps that may be set up very quickly in the first interchanges—traps that can lead the therapist to negate the abilities of the adolescent. If the therapist can avoid such pitfalls and find ways to highlight competence and mastery, he or she can produce dramatic and rapid change in the family system. But the starting place is almost always that inevitable hall of mirrors experienced by the family. To move forward, the therapist must quickly break through those mirrors which imprison both the adults and the disabled child.

Ballooning Small but Valid Moments

My work with this family illustrates another important technique, that of ballooning small but valid moments to unbalance the homeostatic mechanism. In this case the small moment turned out to be the key to therapeutic entry. My discovery of the girl's interest in flowers came in response to the simple question, "What do you like to do?" From this beginning I was able to build for the family a whole structure of competence that surprised them. The previous emphasis, on discovering what the girl could not do, simply disappeared.

It was Salvador Minuchin and H. Charles Fishman (1981) who introduced the metaphor "ballooning the small moment." They cautioned, however, that the art of therapy is in knowing what to balloon. In working with a disabled adolescent the art is in picking up on an incident that will reveal true competence. Ballooning can then prove decisive when it provides evidence to challenge the families' reality.

Of course, there are some caveats in using this technique. The therapist must be careful not to provoke false optimism. The proper use of ballooning hinges on clinical accuracy in determining areas of actual competence—areas that will evoke a reciprocal response from the parents and siblings. To choose an inappropriate area would lead instead to a therapy of condescension and would eventually set the family up for defeat and despair. With Ingrid's family we knew we had hit a true chord when the adults responded with laughter and pleasure when the psychiatrist's decrepit plant was introduced. It was obvious to all that in this area the young girl was far more competent than the eminent doctor.

A Therapy of Experience

According to Jerome Kagan in *The Nature of the Child* (1981), "The structure of beliefs about the self and the world that are most resistant to change is called a frame." (p. 9) This family's "frame"—their belief that their daughter was incompetent, helpless, and hopelessly dependent—was changed *in the session*. Moreover, it was changed in a way that was a consequence of structural family therapy. New experiences do produce a change in frame in most circumstances (Kagan 1984). And this tenet, of course, is an important characteristic of this therapy. It is the family's new experience of seeing their daughter as competent that changes the cognitive frame.

The therapist cannot assume that a new experience will occur outside the context of the session. The therapy must *provide* the experience right then and there. In the case of Ingrid's family the experience provided in the session was one of a radical inconsistency. This was one time that the parents were asked to see their daughter not as a disabled child but as a capable young woman. The therapy put forth a view of Ingrid that was totally inconsistent with the parents' usual way of regarding her. An inconsistency like this is not likely to surface spontaneously; the therapist must work with the system to uncover it in the treatment room.

In Ingrid's case the new experience was provided and an initial frame was set for the therapy. Sessions such as these do not, of course, entail the whole of the treatment. The continuing therapy involves amplifying the frame and making sure it is not inhibited. The therapist works with both the family as a whole and in subsystems to stabilize new structures and thereby maintain change. During this second stage of the therapy the therapist concentrates on not allowing the system to revert back to its denial of the adolescent's strengths.

Ingrid had been in the hospital for two months. In the next sequence I bring up the specter of what will happen when she leaves the hospital.

DR. FISHMAN: How long are you going to be here?

(*There is no response.*)

DR. FISHMAN: The rest of your life?

(*Ingrid shakes her head vigorously in the negative.*)

DR. FISHMAN: Two years?
INGRID: No!
(*loudly and emphatically*):
DR. FISHMAN: One year?
INGRID: No!

Before we could get Ingrid out of the hospital we first had to reinforce her self-confidence. One way to do this was to reemphasize her areas of competence and then challenge her to take on the unknown future. Once her competence was recognized, I could move on. I began by utilizing the old ploy of exaggeration, asking her if she planned to remain in the hospital for the rest of her life. She was immediately motivated to say no, which is what I wanted. Through further questioning I got her to negotiate down the time she would remain in the hospital. The therapeutic art here involved seizing the moment and building on realized competence, so that Ingrid could feel, "I can change things. I am competent. I can make decisions about my life."

Frequently the most difficult part of therapy with disabled adolescents is to get all of the principal helpers pulling in the same direction. In this adolescent's world the sources of feedback are many. The adolescent hears from family, physician, teachers, and other helpers. These divergent sources of response can make it difficult to maintain a positive progressive atmosphere. It may take only one negative source to set back the course of treatment. The therapist must therefore work to include as many of the helpers as possible in reinforcing the adolescent's new identity of self.

A fable comes to mind that I think may help illustrate the reinforcing powers of the outside context. A man coming out of the woods is very, very hungry. He goes into the camp and puts a little stone in a pot. Somebody approaches and asks, "What are you making?" He answers, "Stone soup." The second man tastes it and says, "Well, it's tasting good but it would be better with onion." So he goes and gets an onion. Eventually, each member of the community supplies another ingredient—celery, tomatoes, carrots, and so on—until in the end the first man just removes the stone. Ingrid's "stone" was the plant. The object of the therapy was to get people to rally around her emerging competence. We began with her mastery of plants, and around this fact the family progressively organized and reinforced the idea that the girl was capable in some areas. In the end it did not matter that her capability in handling plants might be a minor issue: the point was that the family had accepted this small capability as a new reality and had begun dealing with her in a variety of other ways as competent and worthwhile.

DR. FISHMAN: Where will you go when you leave the hospital?

(*The mother points to herself.*)

DR. FISHMAN: Congratulations—do you want her at home? Do you want your lovely, grown-up daughter to be at home?
MOTHER: She can't leave. She can't do important things.
INGRID: She's right.
DR. FISHMAN: I don't understand. You know a foreign language but you can't boil an egg—you can't cook at all?
INGRID: I can but only a little. Really.

This sequence represents the second stage of the therapy, where the emphasis is on stabilizing change and preventing a reversion to old patterns. When the therapy is going well it begins with an honest challenge to provoke a new response, one that is inconsistent with the parents' (as well as the adolescent's) belief that the adolescent is incompetent. By amplifying this inconsistency I managed to get Ingrid to say "I can" and her parents to acknowledge, with some reluctance, this new fact regarding their daughter's competence. Now came the ultimate test: stabilizing the change. The goal was for Ingrid to free herself from an institutional dependency. I asked Ingrid, "Where can you go where you will be more autonomous and competent?" At that point it was clear that Ingrid could go anywhere she wished. (I should note that leaving home for a disabled child is a different proposition in Sweden than it is in the United States. In Sweden there are many state-sponsored group homes that can serve as midway places for stabilization prior to the final launch from the family.)

In this family we saw a rising resistance to Ingrid's leaving. The mother's overprotective assumption was that her daughter must return home. I chose to act perplexed, as if I could not understand the mother's assumption. I did this in order to evade resistance. The mother did not mention a place for Ingrid; rather, she pointed to her own body as the girl's destination. I interpreted this as a real sign of pathology, but instead of giving the mother a strange look I congratulated her on the fact that the girl was coming home to her. It was then that I professed my bewilderment about the mother's claim that the girl was incapable and so could not go anywhere else but home.

I believe at that point that the therapy was progressing well. The therapists were meeting the specific obstacles—the specific resistances to the release of the young woman. This was the family's way of keeping the daughter in check. We could now work to change this pattern and help to free the girl. Of course, the parental response with a retarded adolescent in this situation is understandable; the mother and father, with mother as spokesman, were afraid that their daughter would fail—that she would not be able to live on her own. It was almost habitual for this mother to rush forth to protect her daughter by holding her in place. But while the motive itself may have been benign, the practical result would have been anything but: the girl would have been prevented from taking her first steps toward autonomy.

Of course, what was at work in this family system was a kind of inertia. We were less concerned with the dark undercurrents in the mother's behavior, her unconscious attempts to curtail her daughter. As therapists we were more concerned with the surfacing of a system, the homeostatic sequences that emerged when the system was perturbed and that acted to return things to the status quo. The parents and Ingrid had both been challenged to behave differently, yet they had no experience in carrying out the new behavior. The developing patterns allowing change and growth had not stabilized, so the parents were unaccustomed to dealing with any possibility of independence. Their most available response was to jump into action to stop their daughter's flight. The system's inertia stood in the way of the therapist's goal of emancipating the young woman.

The challenge, then, was to find ways both to amplify the moves toward autonomy and, at the same time, to defuse resistance.

| INGRID: | I'm not interested in moving out. |
| DR. FISHMAN (*looking at the mother*): | You know why your daughter is not interested in moving out––because you are such a good cook. |

The task here was to signal the parents that they are blocking autonomy and independence, and to do so without offending them. My way of accomplishing this was to find an innocuous way to suggest that they are hindering their daughter's growth through their benevolence. I gave many such messages to get my point across. This approach worked better than simply declaring the mother an intrusive, overprotective force, because it kept the parents on my side as well as on the side of their daughter. In addition, I knew that any attack on the parents would have made it more difficult for Ingrid to leave. (It is hard, after all, to leave someone who is hurting.) The chosen technique then, was meant to maintain a light tone and to give the mother the message that she is so good to her daughter that she is holding her back.

DR. FISHMAN (*to the mother*):	Are your other children married?
MOTHER:	Two of them are married.
DR. FISHMAN:	Do you hope she gets married one day?
MOTHER:	There's always a hope, but I'm skeptical.
DR. FISHMAN:	Why? (*To Ingrid:*) The boys don't like you?
INGRID:	I don't like them.
DR. FISHMAN:	Oh, that's different. You know what I think interferes with you getting married?
INGRID:	What?
DR. FISHMAN:	Because your parents make it so comfortable for you at home. Because your parents are confused; they don't know what you can do, that you can be more independent.
MOTHER:	There is a problem that she doesn't know how to spell and how to write. There is also the economics—she can't manage economics. We keep her money; we give her some every week.
DR. FISHMAN:	Do you like that?
INGRID:	What?

DR. FISHMAN:	That your mother and father have all your money.
INGRID:	It's best.
DR. FISHMAN:	Why?
INGRID:	I don't know enough about it.
MOTHER (*to the father, in an apparent revelation*):	It might be interesting to give her her money to see how she could do. '
FATHER:	Maybe.
DR. FISHMAN:	I think that's a good idea. See, maybe she's smarter than you think.
FATHER:	Yes, I don't think there's much to be lost. It's worth a try.
MOTHER:	It's a good situation, because if she can handle her money, she can also blow what she wants. It would be interesting to see.

(*While the parents are discussing the possibility of her managing her money, I get up and walk over to Ingrid. I kneel next to her and touch her arm.*)

DR. FISHMAN:	Your mother and father think that you're younger than your age and that you can't handle money. Is that true, or do you want to try? You know English, and you know about plants—why can't you handle money?
INGRID:	No, I don't know English.
DR. FISHMAN:	But you understand me.
INGRID:	Yes.
DR. FISHMAN:	Your mother says you will just spend all your money, but I'll bet you can *not* spend all your money and can prove them wrong.

(*Ingrid looks at me and smiles.*)

DR. FISHMAN:	If you can handle money you can live on your own. Because we know you can cook some things, and we know you know English, and we know there is an area where you can get a job. Then you can live on your own. (*Looking at the mother:*) Would you let her move out?
FATHER (*shaking his head*):	No.
DR. FISHMAN (*to the mother*):	Would you?

MOTHER:	Yes. If she can manage her finances.
DR. FISHMAN:	Maybe she should stay with you for many, many years.
MOTHER:	That's her problem, we can't live her whole life for her. When she moved out, she tried living with people her own age and it didn't work (*shaking her head vigorously*). But then again, it was very close to home and it was easy to go home.
DR. FISHMAN:	Maybe it shouldn't be so easy to go home.
MOTHER (*nodding her head vigorously in agreement*):	We discussed that it was too easy for her to go home and also [that] she was the only girl there. Now there are three more girls there.

The parents turned to one another and discussed the options raised. They agreed that they would first give Ingrid the chance to manage her money and then, if that were successful, allow her to move out into a sheltered situation.

THE FOLLOW-UP

Two weeks after the last session Ingrid was discharged from the hospital and the parents took responsibility for her charge. Ingrid really wanted to go to school, and shortly thereafter she did start going to a school away from home, an intern school where she stayed overnight. In addition, she started taking care of her own money and managed very well, without any failure. During Ingrid's absence the therapists received several telephone calls from the mother, who was frightened about the girl being given too much freedom. She was reassured that Ingrid was doing well and that the course of action taken was absolutely necessary.

The following summer Ingrid got a summer job as a gardener's assistant. For the first time in her life she received an actual salary, not a pension. Later, she went on a vacation with her parents for two weeks. This turned out to be a "disaster," according to her parents. Ingrid kept testing the parents' limits and went out with boys. When the family came back, the mother phoned the therapists again to talk about this new behavior. Again she was reassured that these actions were developmentally in order, and the therapists further complimented her on giving her daughter freedom.

Eventually Ingrid enrolled in an art school, where she also was able to improve her reading and writing skills. She hoped to secure a job as a gardener or as a gardener's assistant. She had a boyfriend, who she met in the new school, and she was very fond of him. Ingrid had not been at home in the last two months and had had no psychiatric breakdown; nor had she required any medication.

Summary

For three years after this consultation I felt very good about the outcome of this therapy. Any time I spoke with Olaf Ulwan, the psychiatrist who headed the clinic in Sweden where the therapy took place, he had regards to me from Ingrid—things like, "Tell Dr. F. that I am doing well and I am very much enjoying my work."

Last year Dr. Ulwan left the clinic and a non-systemic model of therapy was adopted there. Thus, when Ingrid experienced a new crisis (she broke up with her boyfriend and became very depressed) she was hospitalized for an extended period and then sent home to her parents. Apparently, she was neither working nor seeing her friends.

Hearing this news reminded me of some sobering realities about families and family therapy. We must have respect for the chronicity of the previous homeostasis as well as for the nature of the presenting disability. Ingrid and her family were a very stable system with much chronicity in the dysfunctional organization. Her particular disability, retardation, tends to have the power to organize people to be overly helpful. I believe that family therapists should be cognizant of the fact that systems not only transform but they also *transform backward*. Therapists should, with very chronic cases, make provision for this fact, such as asking families to return for regular follow-up interviews. This would help to maintain the new organization of the family system as well as to let the family know that in this "General Practitioner approach," if a new problem emerges, there is someone available to help. If such an arrangement had been in place in Ingrid's family system, chances are that the original therapeutic team would have been able to head off the new crisis.

PART III

TREATING DISTURBANCES OF SUBSYSTEMS: CLINICAL CASES

9

A Single-Parent Family: A Disorganized Organized System

Does my sassiness upset you?
Why are you beset with gloom?
'Cause I walk like I've got oil wells
Pumping in my living room.

Just like moons and like suns,
With the certainty of tides,
Just like hopes springing high,
Still I'll rise.
—MAYA ANGELOU

IN a 1981 presentation at the Philadelphia Child Guidance Clinic, Virginia Goldner discussed the popular notion that "the family is falling apart." Her conclusion was that it is not the *family* that is falling apart, but the concept of the family as the perfect "Ozzie and Harriet" system—the conventional, white, middle-class, two-parent, one-worker couple that marries early, rears children, and does not divorce—that had disintegrated. Goldner's contention is that the contemporary concept of the nuclear family was, in fact, seen as the norm only for middle-class couples that began their households in the first decades following World War II. She asserts that many of the trends cited as proof of the decline of the family, such as declining marriage and fertility rates and rising divorce rates, were actually the norm until the post-war period. This contention is supported by Michael Rutter (1980), who points out that the fertility rate was falling steadily into the 1930s, that the divorce rate has been rising since the late nineteenth century, and that the trends toward later marriage and a higher proportion of the population entering marriage date only from the end of World War II.

It seems clear then, that the stresses on the modern family have been in operation for some time and do not represent significant new information for the therapist. Indeed, as Jane Howard (1978) proposes, the real news is not that families are dying but that they are changing in size and shape. Of fifty-six million U.S. families, Howard reports that only 16.3 percent are of a conventional, nuclear variety. Furthermore, the number of children living in a single-parent household has been variously stated at from 20 to 50 percent of all families; and of these single-parent households most are likely to be headed by separated or divorced women (Hogan 1983).

This change to the single-parent household is a significant reordering of the American family system. As family therapists we need to guard against the prejudice of calling single-parent families "nonintact." The truth is that single-parent families are just as intact as two-parent families, and their needs are not met by treating the members of such a system as individuals who live in a transitional organization. In our practices we will find that the single-parent family is indeed a norm. Treating such a family, however, requires a special use of self by the therapist.

General Principles

CONFIRMING THE PARENT'S SENSE OF SELF

The person *of the parent* comes before the person *as the parent*. This means that the therapist must confirm and reinforce the sense of self of the presiding parent. Self-respect is the key to effectiveness as a parent. For the therapist, then, the priority is to focus first on the parent as an individual. Only when self-respect is confirmed and strengthened is it possible to move on and establish the parent's effective role in the family.

APPLYING THE THERAPIST'S USE OF SELF

The therapist's use of self to support the parent is even more important in working with single-parent households than it is with two-parent families. In many single-parent systems there is no corroboration or support for adult views. The parent, most often the mother, can come to feel outnumbered and overwhelmed and begin to doubt her own sense of what is correct or appropriate. What the therapist aims to accomplish in such situations is to provide options and support for the parent, confirming her view of reality. This process of confirmation can help the individual begin to see herself differently as a person and head eventually to a role change. Frequently the therapist needs to be involved in creating a therapeutic subsystem, albeit an artificial one, in which the therapist supports the parent. By working with the parent it is possible to put together a coherent generational subsystem. This process is crucial because there are fewer options and resources for the single parent.

SEARCHING FOR SUPPORT IN THE LARGER CONTEXT

The third principle for treating single-parent families is that the therapist needs to be even more sensitive to the contemporary forces in the ecology. This heightened sensitivity is essential because the therapeutic subsystem is both temporary and artificial and has less enduring power. It is important, therefore, that the therapist search the larger context to find other individuals, organizations, or institutions that can provide additional support.

Clinical Case: Ruth, Struggling to Please Everybody

The case that follows illustrates many of the challenges presented by a single-parent system. At the time of intervention the mother and her children were in crisis. The mother said the kids were uncontrollable. The mother and father were fighting long-distance over the telephone and the entire system was reverberating from the imminent departure of the eldest daughter for college.

ASSESSMENT USING THE FOUR-DIMENSIONAL MODEL

History

The mother, Ruth, was a single parent who had been divorced for quite some time. The father was not around, having moved to another state. There were four, very attractive children: Hope, age eighteen, Lisa, seventeen, Robert, fifteen, and Jane, twelve. The family had a somewhat unusual living situation in that the mother, in addition to her clerking job, was raising dogs (thirteen at the time) in order to earn money for the kids to go to college as well as to provide for their other needs. It was this living situation that the father found untenable, claiming he could not handle the kids plus all the dogs. Before leaving he had often expressed his rage by severely beating both his wife and the animals.

It was the oldest child, Hope, who contacted the therapist. She was going off to college on a full scholarship and was concerned about leaving the other kids with mother. She raised the possibility of foster care and other alternatives and asked of the therapist, "How can I get my siblings out of the house because Mom is so horrendous?" As an example she cited the plight of the youngest child, who had some goldfish which she loved. When the child misbehaved, the mother threw out the fish food and let the goldfish die.

The mother worked as a payroll clerk and made twenty-two thousand dollars a year. In addition, she received child support. According to Hope, the other girls worked as janitors to pay their tuition in Catholic school because their mother gave them nothing.

Development

Hope was the mother's lieutenant and functioned as a parental child. She had responsibility without true authority. This daughter was strikingly beautiful, with dark eyes and long black hair down to her waist; she was a brilliant student and had been offered a scholarship at an Ivy League school. This move would be an even greater stress for the family since the mother's best support would be far away. This acute pressure emerged against the backdrop of three other adolescents in the home, a major developmental stress even without Hope's leaving.

The mother and father, of course, had developmental issues of their own, including the real-life financial pressures of supporting four increasingly expensive children.

Structure

This system was characterized by an extreme problem in family hierarchy. As the sole representative of her generation in the home the mother did not have her adult perceptions reinforced in the current system; furthermore, father actively undermined her. Her plight typifies that of many a single parent. The children capitalized on their mother's weakness by threatening to live with their father if she attempted to discipline them.

Her inability to deal with such threats had made her more of a peer than an executive to her children. This lack of effective control led to a chaotic home life, which was exacerbated by the mother's overinvolvement with the dogs she was breeding. As with her children, she was incapable of setting limits for the animals and allowed them the run of the house. The resulting chaos had been instrumental in the father's abandoning the family. The continuing animosity between the parents had also been exploited by the children, who played one adult against the other.

Process

From the perspective of the outsider this system was in chaos, lacking even the most rudimentary rules of decorum. At any point, seemingly at random, conflict might erupt and dissolve any semblance of effective control. It was clear that this lack of control was a direct result of the mother's inability to exert executive leadership. Furthermore, the overt conflict among the siblings was commensurate with the considerable conflict avoidance in the mother. She simply was not able to confront her children in a manner that would change their behavior.

As a consulting therapist, my immediate subjective experience on encountering this system was one of extreme anxiety and impotence. The family's constant bickering made me want to run for cover, and my attempts to establish some order or control left me feeling powerless. No sooner had one fire been put out when another would erupt in a completely unexpected area. Moreover, the system exerted a constant pressure on the therapist to be drawn in and take the place of the missing parent. The challenge in the face of this pressure was to continue working to support and bolster the mother's executive authority instead of acting to fill the vacuum and take over for her.

THE HOMEOSTATIC MAINTAINER

In this system the homeostatic maintainer may well have been the father. When things heated up and the mother attempted to exert any authority, the specter of father as an alternative emerged and the mother was defeated. Apparently, the father did not intervene to support his wife, but instead criticized her, even from a distance, and told the children they could come and live with him. In addition, despite the fact that the father had been gone for some time, the mother still harbored a hope that he would return or that somehow they would get back together. This hope reinforced her inaction. Waiting for the father's return was like "waiting for Godot": it kept the mother from facing reality and coming to terms with an unacceptable status quo.

THE THERAPY

The primary goal in the brief therapy with this family was to join with the mother, to create a transitional adult-adult support system that would enable her to function as an effective parent and maintain a workable hierarchy. The therapist's first job was to reinforce the mother's sense of dignity and help her enact a sense of indignation and justification for making difficult but necessary decisions. In the session that follows my focus was initially on attempting to work with the family's therapist to sort through the discord and discover the best way of supporting the mother.

The therapist, a young woman, had seen the family three times. According to the therapist these sessions had been quite unusual, with individuals crying or laughing for no apparent reason. In spite of what the children said, the therapist reported that the mother had spent money for their braces, saw to it that they did their homework, and in general did make an attempt to see to their needs. This woman worked very hard and was not present in the home very much. Her absence, and the fact that there were thirteen dogs with the run of the house, had resulted in an environment that was a shambles.

The session began in relative chaos. It was clear from the beginning that there was an attenuated hierarchy in the system and that there was an extreme amount of overinvolvement and overprotectiveness. Furthermore, the mechanisms maintaining the homeostasis were readily apparent. One of the most powerful of these was the mother's paralysis when the children threatened to go live with their father if she did not accommodate to them. Guilty over the divorce and her part in it, the mother would retreat, saying that she believed it essential for the family to stay together. She could not act in any adult, executive fashion that might carry the risk of dissolution.

In the early part of the session it became clear that the young family therapist had become inducted into the system and was taking the children's side against the mother. I therefore called her out of the room and suggested that she side with the mother, to create a subsystem of therapist and mother, a generational boundary that would help reestablish a functioning hierarchy in the system. What follows is a segment of the session subsequent to that point.

THERAPIST (*to the mother*):	You're trying to please your kids.
MOTHER:	I have been lately. I told them, since the divorce, we're a team. We're supposed to work together.
THERAPIST:	What do you need from them?
MOTHER:	Cooperation. I want them to pitch in and do their share and what I've got right now is blatant rebellion. Every time I open my mouth, it's "Shut up, bitch" from him (*indicating Robert*). We walked out the other day from a counseling session and he stood out by the parking lot and said, "Are you four bitches coming?" I mean, that's not a very good attitude. That's not cooperative. "I have to live with three bitches." He called everyone a bitch all the way home.
THERAPIST:	And what did you do?
MOTHER:	I just figured let him get it out of his system.
THERAPIST:	Do you like being called a bitch?
MOTHER:	Of course not, but I'm not going to cry over it.
THERAPIST:	How about stopping it? You've done a lot, you've come a long way, you've sacrificed a lot in raising these bright, well-put-together kids. And you don't deserve to be called a bitch.
MOTHER:	I know.
THERAPIST:	Does she?
ROBERT:	Yes.
THERAPIST:	Well, I'm sorry, but you're wrong. She's your mother, and mothers don't deserve to be called bitches.

I have a sense that in spite of the intervention, entropy is setting in and the therapist is losing her capacity for therapeutic leadership.

JANE:	He [Robert] says he's been trying to do his share around the house, but he hasn't done one thing.
ROBERT:	You haven't done anything either.
JANE:	Yes, I have . . .
ROBERT:	You guys want me to say my feelings? Fine. I said them all other times—it's getting worse and worse every single time. I didn't do anything to her [the mother].

HOPE: And she [the mother] sits there! This isn't how she is at home! She sits down talking to you [the therapist]—that's not how it is at home. And then you say, "Yes, I think she's a very good mother." Well, I don't think she's a good mother!

LISA: Hope, she's changed.

THERAPIST: How did you get to be valedictorian. . . .

It is evident that there is a coalition of the children against the mother. One against many is a common plight of the single parent. However, the therapist allows herself to be inducted into filling the executive vacuum in the system. She steps in to take over for the mother rather than encouraging her to assert her executive role. By doing so the therapist gives the family the implicit message that the mother is not able to fulfill her parental function.

THERAPIST: How did you get to be where you are without having a very good mother?

HOPE: I had a lot of nice friends.

THERAPIST: Friends don't raise you.

HOPE: Yes, they did, my friends raised me.

THERAPIST: No, this woman raised you.

HOPE: No, she didn't! She didn't raise me. She goes to work and . . .

ROBERT: Bull!

LISA: She did give you food.

HOPE: We've been on our own.

THERAPIST: Mothers raise their children.

JANE: And she pays for haircuts.

HOPE: Maybe she raised me, but she hasn't given me any love.

THERAPIST: What about your braces? Mothers who don't care don't give their kids braces.

ROBERT: Then she shouldn't have given me braces.

HOPE: She didn't give me any braces.

THERAPIST (to the mother):   What do you want from them? You need to let them know what you need. And I will help you get it.

The therapist has been inducted into becoming the mother's champion. In so doing she has rendered the mother even less effective.

MOTHER: First of all, I have raised them to be very independent and self-sufficient. And now they are all so independent and self-sufficient that they are butting heads with me.

THERAPIST: But you are the mother. You need to be the fearless leader.

HOPE: She's never been the fearless leader.

THERAPIST: Well, then I don't know how you got to be where you are.

HOPE: I always had to be the one to take care of them. All my life. Ask any one of them.

ROBERT: Yep.

HOPE: I'm the leader! I did everything! The clothes! I cleaned the whole goddam house! And you say she's the fearless leader. I don't like that. I was the leader.

THERAPIST: No. She's the mother. And the mother is always the leader.

ROBERT: She brought home the bacon, but we fried it.

THERAPIST: If she didn't bring home the bacon, you'd have nothing to fry; just an empty pan. (*To the mother:*) Tell them what you need from them.

MOTHER: Well, if I had two nights a week when I know they're there and have my permission. . . .

(*All of the children are talking at once, giggling and joking derisively.*)

THERAPIST: These kids don't take you seriously.

(*It had become increasingly evident that the session needed to be redirected, and at this point I entered the room.*)

DR. FISHMAN: Hello, I'm Dr. Fishman, I've been behind the mirror.

MOTHER: How do you do, I'm Ruth, and this is. . . .

DR. FISHMAN: Oh, I don't want to meet them. I have no interest in meeting such disrespectful kids. (*To the kids:*) I understand you're even supposed to be bright.

HOPE: Yes, I am pretty bright.

DR. FISHMAN: Well, you'd never guess it. (*To the mother:*) The kids are so disrespectful to you.

MOTHER: That's why we're here. It's come into full bloom in the last two months.

DR. FISHMAN: You don't deserve it.

MOTHER: Thank you.

(When I entered I deliberately sat down next to the mother. She was a moderately overweight woman with brown hair and brown eyes, dressed in slacks and a sweatshirt. As she thanked me I saw her eyes well up with tears.)

DR. FISHMAN:	Why don't you give them a choice? They can stay with you and be respectful and act their ages, or go with their father. You shouldn't have to move and remarry for them. You should have your own life.
ROBERT:	She does.
DR. FISHMAN:	Wait a minute, I'm talking. Your kids probably have a fantasy that you'll get back together and be very happy, but you know there were reasons that you split.
MOTHER:	That has nothing to do with this. But the fact is that I've wanted to go back with him. I talked with him the other day, and we both wanted to do it. But the kids were so terrible—I told them at the time of the divorce that I'd never marry someone if I thought there would be a problem between the kids and that person.
DR. FISHMAN:	Who do they think they are, that they're telling you? Why don't you do this—why don't you have the kids leave, and you and your husband live here.
MOTHER:	Yeah, or I'll go and leave them.
DR. FISHMAN:	That would be a possibility.
MOTHER:	But I can't do that.
DR. FISHMAN:	Sure you can. There are foster homes—if they're not going to be respectful.
ROBERT:	You're just trying to scare us.
DR. FISHMAN:	No, I'm not. I've seen families do it.
MOTHER:	Do you think there's any possibility that this could be solved in some way? That's why we're coming here. That's why I'm bringing us.
DR. FISHMAN:	I don't know, what do you think?
LISA:	I don't want to.
THERAPIST:	I think with all your skills, with all the experience you have, it is a possibility, but you will have to be very strong.
DR. FISHMAN:	I don't know. They treat you like they're your mother, not like you're the mother.
MOTHER:	They tell me what they're going to do and what they're not going to do. We sat down and made jobs, and I'm the only one that's doing mine.

DR. FISHMAN: I don't think they should continue living with you. I think you really should think about that. You're not required by law, you can put them in foster homes. They should earn their keep. The solution is they should earn their keep with you and be respectful to you.

MOTHER: Well, I would never have considered that it was bad enough at this point that that's what I should do.

DR. FISHMAN: Well, talk about it. (*I leave the room.*)

I am attempting to increase the intensity in order to address the important but unstated issues in the system, namely that the mother is being blackmailed by her children's threat to leave and that she is overwhelmed by these demanding adolescents. What is necessary here is, first, to call the children's hand and so remove the power of their threat and, second, to move to support the overwhelmed mother. If we can help the mother take effective and definitive action, even for a short time, it will enhance her position in the system and force the children to accommodate to her rather than her accommodating to them.

As I returned to my position behind the mirror I was hopeful that my intervention would change the course of the session and allow the mother to begin acting on her own behalf instead of relying on the therapist to fill the parental vacuum.

The mother then related a conversation she had had with her ex-husband. As she spoke it became clear that in many ways the children were instrumental in the break-up of the marriage. Apparently, the children would not tolerate their father, and there was a profound coalition of the mother and the children (not to mention the dogs) against the father. In the sequence that follows, the mother is beginning to realize that it may not be possible for them to get back together.

MOTHER: There's too much turmoil, too much agony and hostility. And I said that we couldn't make it because of the kids. And he's willing to wait. Whatever I think is best. He's not going to interfere. He doesn't just want to take Robert and Lisa, and then Hope would go away to college and Jane would be alone while I'm at work. He thinks that would be sad. So he's thinking of everyone. He wants the family to stay together.

THERAPIST: But maybe the family shouldn't stay together.

LISA: I was thinking of going to a foster home on my own. Because I think it's terrible at home. I was thinking about doing it just. . . .

THERAPIST: Maybe that's the best idea.

JANE: I don't want to go.

THERAPIST: You want to stay?

JANE: Yeah, I want the whole family to stay together and be happy. Hope and Lisa are—no, they don't want to—Lisa wants to go to Kansas. If she really wants to go to Kansas, she'll go. Like I said to Mom, "Why don't you just let Hope go, and the rest just stay home?"

MOTHER: What I want is to do what's best for the whole family. And right now we are a family and your father is the long-distance member of the family, but he has a very low tolerance level. He would be totally frustrated, and it would be very difficult for him to handle a situation like this.

THERAPIST: It would be difficult for anyone to handle a situation like this.

MOTHER: He couldn't cope with it. I mean he would be knocking heads against walls. And he would be yelling at me because he usually takes things out on me. But he wants to help me, he doesn't want to see me handle it alone.

The mother's statement that the father does not want her to handle the situation alone corroborates my feeling that this woman looks for people to become her champion. In the absence of the father she inducts the therapist into assuming that role. Of course, her need for a champion to defend her against the children is not a sound reason to reunite with her husband. If the parents decide to reunite it should be from a position of strength, not because the children present such dire problems that a parental coalition is necessary. If they were to pull together just to cope with the children it would be a short-lived relationship, since in any case the children will be gone from the home in a few years. Moreover, it would be a profound boundary violation for the parents to base a reconciliation on the desires of the children.

THERAPIST: What do you want?

MOTHER: Forgetting him—I would like to have a cooperative, helping family without all this hostility between all the different members. The issue of the dogs came up. They all have their favorite dogs, and they use the dogs to irritate each other. If Lisa is mad at Robert, she'll kick his dog. They don't like Jane's dog, so they'll scream at it. They don't like certain dogs because they represent certain people they're mad at.

THERAPIST: It sounds like you have a bunch of kids, and this is how they get at each other. It sounds like you're talking about little kids.

MOTHER: Maybe it's the fact that she [Hope] was only thirteen when we divorced.

LISA: That's a possibility.

THERAPIST: That would be sad. It would be a shame if you were all stuck being kids for the rest of your lives.

LISA: Well, we were raised by a kid—so we're stuck being kids.

THERAPIST: No, you were raised by a woman. It seems to me that if your kids would like you and your ex-husband to get together, if they want to be a family again, they need to prove it to you by showing you that they can work together and be a family.

ROBERT: We don't want to, though. We don't want to. Hope doesn't want to, I don't want to, and do you (*to Lisa*) . . .

LISA: What?

ROBERT: Want Mom and Dad to get together again—and move down there?

LISA: I want them to do what's right—what they'd be happy about and what we'd be happy about.

HOPE: I said to Mom last night, "If you want to go back to Dad then you should go back to Dad." And I mean that. If you really want to go, then go. And forget about us. He should be your first choice. But I also said that I wish she would consider us, and if she does consider us, she won't do it.

THERAPIST: You need to prove to her that she should consider you.

LISA: I said to her on the phone, "Don't even think about us, do what is right for you." That's what I said.

HOPE: That's what I said, too. But she said she's going to consider it. And I'm glad she's considering it. But if she's going to, then . . .

THERAPIST: Wouldn't it be nice if you guys would consider her? Your mother is in the position of having to constantly defend herself.

The therapist is again getting caught up in the role of the mother's champion.

LISA: So are we.
ROBERT: So are we.
THERAPIST: How do you show her?
HOPE: I've been keeping up with the list of things.
ROBERT: So have I.

(*Later in the session the therapist presses the point of changing the children's behavior.*)

THERAPIST   If you investigate foster care and do what needs to be
(*To the*   done to make the children respect you—because they act
mother):   like little children.
ROBERT: If that's what you want—fine.
THERAPIST: That's all I see. That's what you show me.
ROBERT: Whatever. I'm leaving. (*He leaves the room.*)
THERAPIST: You have a very hard task.
JANE: He does that all the time at home, and then there's nothing she can do. What is she going to do, chase him? She locks him out and the front door's broken.

Robert, who had run from the therapy room, was discovered at the end of the day sitting in the waiting room looking very forlorn. The therapist attempted to contact his mother without avail. The family lived in the distant suburbs, about an hour or so away; the therapist transported him for this interim period to a local house for foster children. The foster home was then able to contact the mother and arrange for Robert to be picked up. During the ride home he was screaming at his mother and calling her a "bitch." The mother stopped the car and told the boy to get out. Many hours later, a very contrite son came to the mother's door, apologized and asked if he would be allowed to stay.

For a time things seemed to improve. However, the children eventually reverted to their threat. The mother took them up on it and told them that if they did not shape up they would have to go live with their father. As a result, Robert and Lisa did in fact leave for their father's household.

THE FOLLOW-UP

Following up a year and a half later, I found that the father had turned out to be a terrible caretaker. His twenty-year-old girlfriend lived in the house, he was never there, and the children were neglected. However, Lisa had acquired a boyfriend in the area and so chose to remain with her father. Robert, on the other hand, returned to live with his mother and is now reported to be doing very well, even stating that he "gets along great with Mom."

As for the mother, at one point she was prepared to go through with a reconciliation with her ex-husband. However, at the last minute he called to say he really did not think it would work out after all. Naturally, this was another letdown and was taken as a crushing blow. But the woman was eventually able to begin righting her unbalanced life. She transferred to a less stressful job which allowed her to spend more time at home. And during the absence of the other children she was able to establish a good relationship with her youngest daughter, Jane. In addition, the mother got the house together, reduced the number of dogs to three, and began to build an orderly life out of the chaos. Once she assumed responsibility and established for herself an effective executive role in the family she felt herself to be a bright, competent person able to assert control over what had been an impossible situation.

Of course, this is not a fairy tale, and not every part of the story has a happy ending. Hope, although doing quite well in college, is now completely estranged from her mother. She has become very religious, lives with the family of a friend, and barely speaks to her mother.

Summary

My first impression of this family was from behind a one-way mirror in the observation room. From that vantage point I observed the family enter the room and seat themselves in a semicircle. At first glance it was difficult to pick out the mother. She and three of the children slouched into their chairs, pulling them slightly askew, like rebellious teenagers. In the absolute center of the semicircle, formally dressed and ramrod-straight and attentive, sat the eldest daughter, the parental child. As the session began the therapist, quite naturally, addressed not the mother but this eldest child. I found this scene both poignant and ironic.

This is the occupational hazard that we all fall into at various points in working with systems in which there is a disempowered leader. We find ourselves unintentionally doing exactly what we do not want to do—undermining the very person we should be supporting. The net effect is to disempower that person. This is the same trap that society sets for the single parent, especially when that parent is the mother. The single parent is treated not as the head of an intact system but as a person in transition—awaiting her "other half," a champion, a knight in shining armor. It is the therapist's challenge to avoid that trap.

10

Couples Therapy: The Last Frontier

MAN: Ah, because you would go out tonight . . .
if I could only get inside that
brain of yours and understand what makes
you do these crazy twisted things.
WOMAN: Are you trying to tell me I'm insane.
MAN: That's what I'm trying not to tell myself.
        —CHARLES BOYER and INGRID BERGMAN
           in the movie "Gaslight"

NO BOOK on adolescence would be complete without providing some general principles for the treatment of the parental couple. The core conflict that sustains most family difficulties can be traced to a profound split between the mother and father or other dyads that function as parents. It is therefore extremely important for the therapist to become skillful at probing and modifying the dynamics of the couple, the dynamics that are affecting the stability of the family system.

Therapists often have difficulty treating couples. For the previous generation the mystery was sex. The hope was that if we understood sex, marital discord would be ameliorated. Masters and Johnson and other investigators strove successfully to solve the mystery. We now understand the mystery in a clinical sense and have made available certain applications that have proved great breakthroughs for sexually troubled couples. Why, then, do so many of the couples we see still report having a sex life as barren as the moon, not to mention other problems at least as serious? And why do we have so much trouble treating their complementary angst?

One of the major mistakes that family therapists have made is to address the wrong unit. Carl Whitaker (personal communication, Feb. 1982) says that the individual is only a fragment of the family. I suggest that the couple is, indeed, only a fragment of a larger system and that the significant homeostatic forces that are maintaining the couple's dysfunction must be involved in the therapy at the outset. Once these forces are dealt with and a boundary is created, *then* the couple can exist for therapeutic purposes.

In many cases these significant homeostatic forces are the adolescents whose problems bring the family into therapy in the first place. Treating the couple, then, can be looked at as an essential therapeutic stage in working with the adolescents; indeed, it is not too much to say that this step is in many ways the critical determinant of the outcome of therapy. If the therapy does not deal with this pivotal unit, the therapist cannot be sure that the therapy has been successful, even if the presenting problems of the adolescent have abated.

One might think of the therapeutic approach here as a kind of peeling off of layers. Once an appropriate boundary is created between the parental and adolescent subsystems, the adolescent is liberated, no longer involved in stabilizing and maintaining the family's homeostasis. However, often this liberation also means that the couple is rendered extremely unstable. This process will be evident in the case study later in this chapter.

General Principles

LOOKING FOR "GASLIGHTING"

In the movie *Gaslight* a man, Charles Boyer, tries to convince his wife, Ingrid Bergman, that she is going insane so that he can have her committed. For example, he secretly turns down the gas jets, and when his wife asks if it is getting dark in the room he responds, "No, dear, it must be your eyes. You are imagining things." This subtle, destructive process continues until the wife is indeed convinced that she is going mad. She no longer trusts her own perceptions that confirm her reality.

"Gaslighting" is this process of allowing one's independent perception of reality to give way to the opinions and definitions provided by someone else.

Gaslighting is a destructive pattern commonly seen in couples. If you assume that a functional couple should have equality, then each member should have the freedom to express themselves and be met with respect. Furthermore, each spouse should be able to be both complementary as well as symmetrical to the other. When one spouse is being gaslighted by the other, a perceptual apparatus is being undermined. That spouse cannot respond in a symmetrical way. That spouse cannot challenge and, thereby, negotiate differences. When this is the case, the system becomes rigid and the marriage, at the very least, stagnates.

ADDRESSING THE COMPLEMENTARY AND SYMMETRICAL PATTERNS

Working with couples presents a particular challenge for a therapy that looks to perceive dysfunctional interactional patterns and then to change them in the therapy room. When there are three family members one can look for conflict avoidance being diffused by a third party or for coalitions and relative disengagement. But how do we ascertain whether change has, in fact, occurred in couples therapy?

One way of gauging change is provided by Gregory Bateson's concept of symmetrical and complementary sequences. According to Bateson (1979), there are essentially two kinds of behavioral interactive sequences: one is a symmetrical sequence or competition, like a tennis match; the second is a complementary one-up, one-down situation, where one family member nurtures the other or capitulates. What becomes dangerous and pathological in rigid systems is that one pattern or the other becomes fixed and the system moves toward a schismogenesis, a dangerous escalation leading to a breakup of the system.

BRINGING ABOUT REDRESS OF GRIEVANCES IN THE ROOM

Couples therapy needs to involve the redressing of grievances in the room. The couple must be able to forgive each other for the sins of the past. It is a kind of public ritual that will allow them to go on. In cures done with torture victims, the victims always say, "Let me tell you what happened to me." They require witness to their pain, so that it can be acknowledged and a cure can be allowed to happen. This is the essential process of redressing grievances. The systemic issue here is justice. Getting things right and even allows the couple to confess and to forgive and to move on. It is lancing the boil so that healing can occur.

UNBALANCING

In working with couples, the most powerful therapeutic technique is unbalancing—the differential use of the therapist's self to side with and take distance from different spousal members. Unbalancing creates a powerful experience when one spouse sees the other supported by the therapist. It forces the unfavored spouse to see the other with renewed respect. On the other hand, it renders the supported spouse a different sense of self. Through unbalancing the therapist creates an experience that addresses the customary perceptions and forces reevaluation. In the session to follow, the unbalancing was done by consecutively supporting and distancing from each spouse. In so doing it created a cascading intensity.

Clinical Example:
Dorothy, Gaslighted for Twenty Years

ASSESSMENT USING THE FOUR-DIMENSIONAL MODEL

History

In this family we are dealing with a typical "adolescent" problem, anorexia, but here the patient is not the child but the mother. Dorothy had been anorexic since college, a period of more than twenty years. The problem had first emerged when her intrusive parents interfered in what Dorothy described as the most important relationship she had had with a young man up to that time. Somehow her father had called the man, making some accusations regarding pregnancy, and the relationship had been terminated.

During the course of the subsequent anorexia Dorothy took huge amounts of laxatives. The laxatives disequilibrated her blood chemistry, and at least five times she was rushed to the hospital in a coma. (Interestingly, on these occasions the etiology of her comas was never diagnosed.) At the start of therapy Dorothy was five feet, seven inches tall and weighed seventy pounds. Her husband, Herb, was a successful lawyer. They had two children, Greg, age sixteen, and Jenny, age twelve. This was the first psychotherapy the family had attempted.

Greg and Jenny are both morose youngsters. They felt sad most of the time and inadequate around their peers. They tried spending time with their friends; however, they felt guilty about being away from home. They said that they had great difficulties concentrating at school because they were so worried about what was happening at home, especially with their mother's illness.

Development

There were a number of potentially destabilizing developmental pressures in the system. There were two adolescent children, who were being pulled by their peers and their schools to spend time away from home. Dorothy's parents were in their mid-sixties, retiring, and would have more time to spend at Dorothy's home. This added time with her parents served to exacerbate both already rocky marriages. For Dorothy and Herb these developmental issues created a time of serious middle-age reassessment.

Structure

Both her parents and her children were inappropriately close to Dorothy. In addition, Dorothy and Herb were distant as spouses. Dorothy's parents had a very conflicted relationship. Each of them would frequently go to Dorothy with their complaints about the other. There was also an alliance between Herb and their son.

Process

This was a classic psychosomatic family. There was an extreme amount of enmeshment, conflict avoidance, diffusion of conflict, triadic functioning, rigidity, and overprotectiveness. It cannot be emphasized too strongly that these parents demonstrated all of the disruptive characteristics of the psychosomatic family.

In the course of therapy, I met with this couple, together with the wife's parents, twice. During both sessions I had to struggle not to get pulled into the role of Dorothy's savior. I liked her very much and felt that the system was robbing her of her self. I constantly had to remind myself that Dorothy was playing her part in the psychosomatic drama. Any attempt on my part to become a crusader for Dorothy would only have made things worse for this troubled wife: the family undoubtedly would have scapegoated her more and I would have been less effective as a helper for the entire system.

As I studied this family it became clear that the homeostatic maintainers for Dorothy's condition were all of the significant people in her life: her husband, her children, and her parents. Any time Dorothy would attempt to challenge the status quo, one of these significant others would disqualify her. For example, her husband would say, "It's all in your mind." When she tried to get outside the system for confirmation—expressing a desire to go to work, for example—her husband or parents would dismiss such notions as impossible.

Successful therapy with this couple depended on the satisfactory completion of other stages of therapy. As noted previously, there were important homeostatic-maintaining influences in the larger context. Dorothy's parents intruded profoundly into her marriage, and her children were also much involved in maintaining the dysfunction. Indeed, each generation intruded into the affairs of the others, and each generation was recruited by the others to stabilize the dysfunctional status quo. What was needed was a therapy of stages. One could deal with the marital couple only when these other intrusive layers had been peeled off. As the outer layers were removed, the couple would be isolated from the larger context and rendered increasingly unstable and therefore open for change.

THE THERAPY

From my assessment of the system I saw that the most dysfunctional dyad—the relationship that was creating the most stress in Dorothy's life—was her relationship with her parents. I therefore began the therapy with two sessions with Dorothy, her husband, and her parents.

Therapy with Dorothy and Her Parents

In our first session Dorothy's father, wearing a plaid jacket, green pants, and an open shirt, had the look of a retired man. Fidgeting, sighing frequently, restless and bored, he fixed his gaze directly on his daughter. Her mother was conservatively dressed, as though for business—a striking contrast to her husband, who seemed dressed for puttering around the house. The seating chosen by the family clearly reflected the structure of the system. Dorothy was sitting much closer to her parents than to her own husband.

Every Sunday throughout their married life Dorothy and Herb had been visited by Dorothy's parents. The parents never said what time they were coming, and Dorothy and Herb never asked. But every Sunday the family waited to eat until the grandparents arrived. In the following sequence I work to help free Dorothy from patterns of enmeshment in her family of origin.

DR. FISHMAN: What are the reasons that you would like to change things? Are there ways in which you want to change things between you and your parents in terms of your relationship?

DOROTHY: I would like to be able to—I'd like to have my cake and eat it too. I'd like to be able to see you when I want to see you and not see you when I don't want to see you. How do you like that?

MOTHER: Does that happen now? Does that happen now?

DOROTHY: How's that for starters?

MOTHER: Does that happen now?

DOROTHY: No. Do you want to know why?

(Dorothy was clearly becoming very agitated, and to calm her I went over to her and shook her hand.)

DOROTHY: Can I do that now? No. Because in my heart I know I won't be the good girl if I don't call and if I don't see you. So therefore, I can't keep perpetuating that behavior.

FATHER: We love Ralph as much as we love you—Ralph doesn't call me on the phone every night. He lives down in New York; he lives his life.

DOROTHY: I would like to be able to see you when I want to see you . . .

MOTHER: Good.

DOROTHY: And not see you when I don't want to see you.

MOTHER: Good.

DOROTHY: And not to feel guilty about it.

MOTHER: Good—it would be great.

DOROTHY: And not have to lie about it—or make excuses—I'm going here, I'm going there, I did this, I did that . . .

Feeling she has my help, Dorothy challenges the enmeshment in the system. This challenge, seemingly so simple, has not happened before.

MOTHER: Okay. Why do I call you on a Sunday and say, "Are you going to be home? Are you doing anything?"

DOROTHY: And I say, "No." Can I just say I don't feel like seeing you today?

MOTHER: Yes, you should just say, "Mother, not today." Why do you have to make up stories like "We're going here, or there, we won't be home."

DOROTHY: Can I just say I don't feel like seeing you today?

MOTHER: Why can't you come out and say, "No, mother"?

DOROTHY: Because that would hurt you.

MOTHER: No it wouldn't!

FATHER: No it wouldn't. Just say, "Look, we have something to do."

DOROTHY: But suppose I don't have anything to do? Sometimes I just don't feel like seeing anybody, that's all.

MOTHER: Say it!

FATHER: Why do you think your mother calls?

MOTHER: Do you think you're putting something over on me—when you do it?

DOROTHY: Yes.

MOTHER: You're not. I always say, "Why make up these stories when I call?"

DOROTHY: Why the hell didn't we talk about this before?

DR. FISHMAN: Why don't you just talk about it now?

MOTHER: That fear to upset you again, that you're not going to eat again. This is why we didn't talk about it, and you know how it would end if we were discussing this at home.

DOROTHY: I don't understand—even with me—why is what I eat of primary importance?

MOTHER: I want you to be nourished.

FATHER: It's your problem.

DR. FISHMAN: It's not a problem—it's a habit.

After this session with the family of origin, disengagement began. Dorothy successfully negotiated for less visiting with her parents, and the hub phenomena were addressed: the enmeshment, the overprotectiveness, the rigidity. What follows is from the second session with Dorothy and her parents.

DR. FISHMAN: Okay, how is everybody?

MOTHER: Good.

FATHER: Good. How've you been?

DR. FISHMAN: Everybody okay?

MOTHER: Great.

DOROTHY: Except for me. They think this is very easy, but it isn't easy for me.

It is a very tense moment. Dorothy takes on the mantle of being the one who is the patient, thereby diffusing the tension.

DR. FISHMAN: How come?
DOROTHY: Yes, it's very hard. It's the most difficult thing I've ever done.

This is important information about the overprotective-ness and the rigidity of this system. Here is a woman who has raised two children to mid-adolescence, and yet the most difficult thing she's ever done is to bring her parents to see a therapist.

DOROTHY: I found something out that I have not known for twenty years. I had evidently blocked things out in my head and created this lie in my own mind, and I was so shocked last week.

As Dorothy was talking I turned to her husband and asked him to move his chair into the session. I was beginning a low-intensity but essential therapeutic move. I needed to clearly bring him in, in order to pull Dorothy out of this family soup. Dorothy was relating the events of twenty years before, when her parents were involved in breaking up her relationship with a young man. My hunch was that the man involved in that relationship was someone who would have challenged the family rules, and that, of course, could not have been tolerated.

DOROTHY: My father told me he never broke up a romance, that my roommates had called and that there was a pregnant girl at college and he had used me. I never knew that. I believed that I had this wonderful romance that was ended. And I knew it, because Mother said, "You got letters from your roommate and you were there when the phone call came through from them." And I honestly don't remember. There are times in that whole block of time I don't remember. They told me some of the things that I did. I wish I could remember it, but I've tried too hard and I can't. It's like they're talking about somebody else. I've created this lie to myself for twenty years and kept telling myself—and that's what I believe.

DR. FISHMAN: I thought you were going to be talking about Sunday mornings.

Rather than mucking about in what happened a generation ago, I want to talk about a problem that is current, a pattern that is currently driving Dorothy—and I think the rest of the family—crazy.

DOROTHY
(*pointing to
her parents*):   They just haven't been there.

FATHER
(*laughing*):   If you feel that way about it, the hell with you.

Although the father offers his response as a joke, his reaction speaks to the rigidity of the system: if you are unhappy with the pattern, then you will be banished, "the hell with you."

FATHER: We were invited to our son's house. We figured we'd better leave them [Dorothy and her family] alone.

MOTHER: Leave them alone, when they're ready I'm sure they'll call and tell us when to come up.

FATHER: I miss my grandchildren. I don't want to give them a guilt complex or anything, but I miss my grandchildren.

Grandfather pulls out the big guns.

DOROTHY: You can come up.

FATHER: It's okay . . .

DR. FISHMAN: No, go ahead, go ahead. You miss your grandchildren a lot.

FATHER: Oh, I see them. They miss me more than I miss them by now.

DR. FISHMAN: It must be really hard on you.

FATHER: No, not really, because we went down to the club and played in the sun and swam for the afternoon. We didn't suffer that much.

DR. FISHMAN: What do you do for Sunday breakfast?

FATHER: I never ate Sunday breakfast at their house (*laughing and pointing at Herb*). I wouldn't steal any of his eggs.

There is a kind of competition between Dorothy's father and her husband. Her father may not want to "steal" Herb's food, but Herb has already stolen something from him: his daughter.

MOTHER: We never came for breakfast. Oh, no, he gets up and does a whole day's work before that. We just don't live like most people. We get up and we work very hard from the minute we get up. And our schedule is kind of different from most people's. We just are very active people, and we just keep doing and doing—and stop when we're ready.

DR. FISHMAN: Well, that's fine. But go ahead, talk more about what you miss about the Sundays.

MOTHER (*to Dorothy*): You said that we came at 12:30 instead of 2:00. And you cut your finger because we came at 12:30.

DOROTHY: Okay, I'll tell you why, because I know he (*indicating Herb*) gets aggravated. I know that it bothers him and so, as a result, I'm like that. Because I don't want you to know that he's annoyed, so that I try to. . . .

Here we see the tragedy of this woman's life for all these years. She is caught between her husband and her parents; she is the wishbone torn between them. When her parents surprised her by coming early, Dorothy had a psychosomatic response and cut her finger.

MOTHER: And like I said—come out with it, "Come up at 2:00," or whatever. I call you every time before we come up. Every Sunday I say, "Are you going to be home?" I think that's probably one of the smaller things.

By calling it a "small thing," the mother is attempting to avoid conflict. For Dorothy to be entrapped with her family every Sunday is hardly a small thing. This is an issue on which Dorothy should hold her ground until it is resolved.

DR. FISHMAN: Don't diminish it. Hold your ground.

HERB: When we go back over things—Dorothy used to get up-
          tight and get all excited—you know, when the kids were
          little. "Fine—come in, wake them up so you can see them
          before you go home"—you know, little things like that.
          The only thing that bothered me was when the kids
          started screaming, not his coming in and looking at them.
          Then the baby was up all night, but he wanted to see
          them.

          This is extraordinary conflict avoidance. Grandfather
          would get the kids so excited that they would be up all
          night, and no one would say, "Stop it, we have certain
          boundaries around our family." What bothered Herb was
          the kids' screaming, not that the grandfather came in and
          got them overexcited.

DOROTHY: But then again he [*Herb*] doesn't object to a whole lot,
          ever. I mean, he does not object to much at all.
HERB: It upset her and got her all excited, and then it got me mad
          or aggravated, because I had to live with her.
DOROTHY: I was getting excited about things that maybe I was imag-
          ining. Maybe they weren't real things to get upset about.

          Dorothy is describing the process of gaslighting. She
          would get upset and the system would tell her, "It's all in
          your mind."

DR. FISHMAN: Like what, what are some things? You mean like the
              Sundays?
DOROTHY: I've been unhappy about too many things, and maybe
          that's my problem. Maybe that was something within me,
          that I shouldn't have been so jumpy and so aggravated
          and hostile. See, I wouldn't take any kind of advice or any
          type of suggestion. I had to do everything my own way.
DR. FISHMAN: Oh, that's not what I'm hearing. I'm hearing that you're a
              person who accommodates to people all the time.
DOROTHY: Yeah, I guess I do.

At my challenge to Dorothy's perception that she always gets her own
way, there was a pause. It was almost as though a shiver went through the
system. I continued to point up their conflict avoidance. When had they
had a conflict—this week? This month? This year? Last year?

DOROTHY:	Just when I thought Pop would come around and say, "You're getting terribly skinny," and I would get so hostile. I mean, it was just like my head would go berserk. I would be so inflamed and aggravated when he would say, "You have to start taking care of yourself, you're getting too skinny," or something to that effect. I would just get so mad, I would just be able to feel I was so mad. Then one time I did yell.
DR. FISHMAN:	Why don't you talk together about areas that you, Dorothy, have avoided.
DOROTHY:	It's very hard for me to talk that way to anybody.
DR. FISHMAN:	Try it now, because it's important.
DOROTHY:	It doesn't come easy for me.
DR. FISHMAN:	That's okay. Nothing important comes easy for people. See, one characteristic of your family, it seems to me, is that everybody is a conflict avoider.
DOROTHY:	Ignore it and it will go away.
DR. FISHMAN:	Everybody seems to thrive on it.
DOROTHY:	What happens when you avoid conflict all the time?
DR. FISHMAN:	Things don't change, and to the extent that things don't change you focus on not eating, on the anorexia.
MOTHER:	For years I've been aware not to upset you in any way. You're trying to think of some conflict that we had. I've been aware of trying to avoid conflict.

Therapy with the Children

The second stage of therapy was with Dorothy, Herb, and the children. In order to work with the internal dynamics of the marriage we needed to get the other dysfunctional relationships that were disequilibrating the couple in order.

It became clear very early on that the children were living a life of fear, the fear that their mother would go into a coma again and that they would not be there to rush her to the hospital. One or the other of the children was always with her, quietly observing her. This preoccupation and the ensuing isolation from peers inevitably stunted the children's development.

Working to free these children from their mother could only be done with the help of the father. He had to be there as co-therapist as the mother and children distanced, not only to support his wife but to provide comfort to the children so that they could get to work on their own developmental needs.

At the first session with the children, Dorothy had many nervous mannerisms and sat very uncomfortably in her chair, as though it were too hard. Her husband, who in contrast to her painful thinness had a small pot belly, was dressed very conservatively. Greg and Jenny were striking in appearance in that both were dressed much older than their stated years and were not wearing any of the trendy, stylish clothes of the adolescent.

DR. FISHMAN:	You're there to keep an eye on your mom.
JENNY:	To keep her company.
DOROTHY:	I didn't know that.
JENNY:	You know I always ask you, "Do you want me to keep you company?"
DOROTHY:	I always tell you, "No—go. I don't want any company."
DR. FISHMAN (to Jenny):	But you know she doesn't really mean it.
DOROTHY:	But I do mean it.
JENNY:	I know. I don't want you to be alone . . .
DOROTHY:	No, I really do mean it. You don't understand that that doesn't bother me at all. I'd rather see you with your friends. I keep telling you, Jenny, I'd always rather see you with your friends.
JENNY:	Well, I don't always want to be with my friends. Sometimes I just feel like staying home.
DOROTHY:	As long as you feel like staying home just to stay home because you feel like it, not so. . . .
JENNY:	I didn't feel like going anywhere. I felt like staying home.
DR. FISHMAN:	Really, she needs you there to take care of her, doesn't she?
JENNY:	Yeah.
DOROTHY:	No, I don't.
GREG:	I always feel guilty about the time she got real sick and I was out—the first time.
JENNY:	I was there.
GREG:	You were there and I wasn't.
DOROTHY (excited):	You feel guilty about that?
GREG:	Yes, because Jenny was there and I wasn't, and you got really sick.
JENNY:	I didn't know what to do.
DR. FISHMAN:	So one of the two of you is always there.
JENNY:	Uh-huh.

GREG:	Chances are if you came to our house at any time one of us would be there.
JENNY:	Or both of us.
DR. FISHMAN *(to Jenny):*	How old are you?
JENNY:	Twelve.
DR. FISHMAN:	Twelve. *(To Greg:)* And you're sixteen?
JENNY:	Like, I walked through the door from school, and I see Mom on the sofa screaming her lungs out. She says, "Call Mrs. Brown. Get her over here." I called her up and all. If I wasn't home, I don't know what she would have done.
GREG:	She couldn't get up or anything.
JENNY:	She couldn't move.
GREG:	If one of us wasn't there you might have died.
DOROTHY:	Oh, no. But that happened so long ago. I made you a promise when I was in here—I said that'll never happen again . . .
DR. FISHMAN:	You don't believe it, do you?
DOROTHY:	They don't, and they have no reason to believe it yet.
DR. FISHMAN:	You see that—your mother just disqualified you.
JENNY:	I believe it.

In order to create increased intensity I utilize the youngsters' report on their mother's eating to highlight the absurdity of their task.

DOROTHY:	I can tell you—all I have to do is eat and it doesn't happen, Jenny.
GREG:	Did you eat today?
DOROTHY:	Yes, I ate today.
JENNY:	Yes, she did, I was there.
DR. FISHMAN:	Did you feed her?
JENNY:	No, no.
GREG:	But we were there to watch.
JENNY:	I mean there's always someone.
DR. FISHMAN:	Were you assigned to her?
GREG:	No, I wasn't.
JENNY:	I was.
GREG:	I didn't get up in time to see you eat breakfast.
DOROTHY:	And Herb watched when we were on vacation. I did a lot better. I have a lot of room for improvement.

I was creating a crisis around the hub phenomena—the children's overprotectiveness and the enmeshment, the inappropriate and diffuse boundaries between the generations that gave the children the responsibility for rescuing their mother, who had a child's symptoms. Another characteristic now apparent was the rigidity of the system. Dorothy had an all or nothing response to being upset. In effect she was saying, "If you upset me, I will kill myself; it's either my way or nothing." Instead of expressing her anger verbally, Dorothy manifested a life-and-death symptom, her laxative abuse. Almost all of her episodes of coma were secondary to conflict, especially conflict with her own parents.

The therapeutic technique I used with Dorothy was unbalancing. From earlier sessions it became apparent to me that I had become quite important to Dorothy. My presence in the therapy room had enabled her to challenge her parents for what appeared to be the first time in many years. In the course of this session with the children I distanced myself from her and challenged her. This mild unbalancing was extremely important, especially in view of the notion that people change for their therapist, particularly in the early stages of therapy. My sense was that Dorothy would change in order to reestablish proximity with me. (This hypothesis was borne out the following week, when the family came in without the children. I congratulated the father for having managed it, but Dorothy interjected that he had nothing to do with it; she was the one who got the youngsters out.)

The session was aimed at breaking the enmeshment. I was searching for a concrete parameter that would embody all of the patterns. If the therapy got the children out of the house, relieving them of their nursemaid role, we would have a sense that it had been at least partially successful. If, however, the work with the couple that followed was not successful, the enmeshed structure that exploited the children would reappear.

If I had tried in this next segment just to bring the mother to cognitive awareness of her relationship to the children, there might have been insight but no concrete demonstration of restructuring. For truly brief therapy, pivotal structural patterns had to change. The only way to have true structured change was to have the husband pull; it was not enough for the wife just to push. By bringing in Herb as co-therapist there would be a natural force in the system encouraging Dorothy to let go of her parents. His pulling would intimate, "I'll be there for you." Finally, after all these years, her husband, who had been like a brother, a nonchallenger of the system, could work to get the son and daughter out. This was a parental task. To underline the enormity of the inappropriateness of their role, I highlighted the waste of adolescent opportunity for growth.

DR. FISHMAN: So, Jenny, how much time a week do you spend?

JENNY: I might say—a lot—fair—three quarters of the time.

DR. FISHMAN: Three quarters. If you get a chance, do you go out with your girlfriends?

JENNY: Oh, yeah.

DR. FISHMAN: Yes, how much?

JENNY: Whenever I want.

DR. FISHMAN: How much is that?

JENNY (*to Dorothy*): How much?

DOROTHY: It's however much *you* want. In other words, it's always a choice.

Dorothy is about to derail the purpose of my query, so I turn back.

DR. FISHMAN: So you can't even remember, you have to ask your mother. When was the last time you went out with a girlfriend?

JENNY: Out? Like out somewhere?

DR. FISHMAN: Went to the mall? I mean, twelve-year-old girls like to go to the mall.

DOROTHY: Were you at Bonnie's yesterday?

JENNY: Yeah.

DR. FISHMAN: Who was home with your mother?

JENNY AND DOROTHY: Dad.

FATHER: And her mother and father.

DOROTHY (*laughing*): That's another story.

DR. FISHMAN: What can you do for these kids to stop this? Because this is all upside down.

DOROTHY: I would like to know how I can get them out of the house. I really mean that. I don't want to get rid of them, but I want them out.

HERB: If you would have something to eat.

DR. FISHMAN: No, the question now is how to get the kids out of the house. You have tried for twenty years to get Dorothy to eat, don't try it here.

The redirecting of the family forces shown in the stark triangle is of pivotal importance. As long as the husband is busy watching his wife, he will not fulfill his parental function, which is to pluck the adolescents away from her. Of significance here is the diagnostic verity that it would be easier to help them fly from her than to make her eat. We must change not the name of her problem, the eating disorder, but instead the troubled context that keeps her from eating: her distant husband, her intrusive parents, and her overly helpful children.

HERB:	Yeah, but isn't that why the kids won't leave the house?
DR. FISHMAN:	No. The kids are in the house because there is somehow an inappropriate job in your house.
HERB:	Well, they're not in any trouble. (*He laughs.*)

> To the father, the children are not in any trouble because they do not make any disturbance.

In this conflict-avoiding family the children do not seem to be in trouble because there is no expression of conflict. They appear difficult to diagnose in that there are few overt signs. But adolescents in this type of existential situation may be destined to become very troubled young adults. An adolescent with no ostensibly defined syndrome can still be heading toward trouble. The preventive task is to analyze their situation and discover whether they are on too short a leash, too curtailed to move on to the next developmental stage. The contextualist, by looking at the way people relate to their immediate context, is less likely to miss adolescents who seem symptom-free but are in the process of becoming problematic young adults. It is important to diagnose not just the adolescent but also circumstances surrounding the adolescent.

DR. FISHMAN:	Yes, they are, because they are missing a lot of important experiences in adolescence that will help them to grow up. There are important types of growth experiences, like the times a twelve-year-old girl has with her girlfriends, that they are not having. Instead you have a couple of practical nurses (*pointing to the children*).
DOROTHY (*to the children*):	I think inside you are both kind of—you know, pooh-poohing this whole idea. You're saying I really do like this.
DR. FISHMAN:	Dorothy, I don't want you to handle it. In other words, they don't have to agree because they both think that you are absolutely irresponsible.

DOROTHY: I know that.

DR. FISHMAN: So how can you make it so that they stop being your mother and father? When we started therapy we had your mother and father come in. I think I might have had the wrong ones. This is your father (*pointing to the son*) and this is your mother (*pointing to the daughter*).

DOROTHY: How can I get them to stop doing this? By not being an adolescent myself. By taking some control over my life.

DR. FISHMAN: Umm. But that's probably unlikely, though.

DOROTHY: You know, I tried last year and I pooped out. But not in that respect. I tried to go to work, and it wasn't fitting in with everybody's schedule, and it just kind of faded by and I . . .

DR. FISHMAN: I don't want to know about that. Do something with the kids right now. Because they shouldn't be there to be your mother and father. It's just not right. Do you agree with me?

DOROTHY: Yes, but I just don't know what to do.

DR. FISHMAN   Because right now your family is upside down. The kids
(*to Herb*):   are mothering Mother, and I don't see Dorothy as changing it. I don't think she wants to. I think she likes having the kids like this.

DOROTHY: I don't like to.

DR. FISHMAN: Otherwise she wouldn't do it. (*To Herb:*) So I'm gonna look to you to change it. You are the only one who can.

HERB: Yeah, but I don't know how to arrange that.

DR. FISHMAN: I don't know either, but I think you need to because Dorothy says all the time, "Well you know, I'm just a poor, poor wet noodle and I can't be responsible," and you're a man of the world. So, in other words it's you who needs to change that. I'm certain of that.

HERB (*shrug-   Well, I guess I'll have to take the kids out of the house
ging and*   myself.
laughing):

DR. FISHMAN: All right, or order them out. I see it as real serious, and I see Dorothy as absolutely not motivated to change it. I mean she talks about eating as if it's the second coming, and it isn't, all she has to do is eat. And so she's not motivated at all. You're the only one who is. Your kids are bright kids and really nice kids, but they don't have the maturity of judgment. So you're the only one who can. I mean, I'm telling it to you as straight as I can.

HERB: Yeah, I'm hearing you but I'm trying to think about what I can do about it.

DR. FISHMAN: You are captain of the ship.

DOROTHY: Can I ask a question?

DR. FISHMAN: No, I'd rather not.

I engage Herb directly, trying to increase his participation by using an image of leadership that has been painfully missing. One would think that Dorothy wants this, but instead she activates to interfere and to try to arrest the participation. I resist the intrusion and pull him out.

DOROTHY: Okay.

DR. FISHMAN: You're the captain of the ship. (*Herb is nodding in agreement.*) It really needs to change, and Dorothy isn't going to budge. And the kids are too concerned in this crazy, upside-down family.

HERB: Well, we're gonna have to start thinking about ways to alter that relationship.

DR. FISHMAN: Don't start thinking about it. Do something. Maybe you want to talk to Dorothy about it, whatever—but I think it should change as of today. Go ahead, what are you going to do? Because it really needs to be done.

Once the father has accepted the role of captain I insist that change begin immediately. As he begins to demand change, the family's resistance can be observed.

HERB: Well, Jenny, you're going one place or the other, right?

JENNY: To Shirley's, if I'm invited.

HERB: Well, we'll get you invited. Okay, that takes care of Jenny.

DR. FISHMAN: For how long?

JENNY: For a week.

HERB: We can't palm her off for more than a week.

DR. FISHMAN: Okay. But what happens when she comes home? I mean, you can't send her to join the Foreign Legion. You're going to have to do something.

JENNY: I don't want to go anywhere.

DR. FISHMAN: See that, she doesn't want to go anywhere. She doesn't have the judgment to know that she's mustn't stay home and be her mother's mother.

JENNY:	But, I want to be—because we have a pool. I mean, why would I want to leave? We have everything I need at home.
HERB:	Yeah, but you'd like to spend a few days with Shirley, wouldn't you?
JENNY:	Uh-huh.
FATHER:	Yeah, well, that will work out.
DR. FISHMAN:	All right, well, that's a start. How about him (*pointing to Greg*)?
DOROTHY:	Greg has been home very little this summer. I'm going to be honest, he really has been going out.
DR. FISHMAN:	See what's gonna happen?
HERB:	He's going to take over for me.
DR. FISHMAN:	See, you're reading me. We're on the same wave length.

> *Family participants routinely perceive the phenomena around them in structural terms. The family therapist seldom has to work hard at imbuing in them a sense of structure. This father immediately sees, "He's going take over for me."*

I have managed to keep the father responding to me as the diagnostician and fixer of his own family. The techniques used to increase the father's participation and centrality were beginning to pay off. He was obviously observing his family acutely and diagnosing correctly the possible shift in forces. He saw that unless he moved, the children would take over for him.

In the sequence that follows the family resists change as the youngsters continue to participate in their mother's eating problem. I work to erode the established pattern.

DR. FISHMAN (*to Greg*):	But you're home for every meal, aren't you? You're watching your mother.
GREG:	Not for every meal. For dinner, Dad's at home.
DR. FISHMAN:	Watching your Mom eat?
JENNY (*interjecting*):	And breakfast.
DR. FISHMAN:	You watch every one of her bites?
GREG:	No, but I see how much she takes all the time.
JENNY:	Yeah, I do.
DOROTHY:	Would they stop watching if I ate more?

DR. FISHMAN: You'd better ask them, I don't know.

DOROTHY (*to Greg*): Let me ask you this.

GREG: If you ate and you were perfectly normal, I don't think I'd care.

DOROTHY: Would you feel better about leaving? If I ate more? Not if I ate more—if I weighed fifteen pounds more?

GREG: Twenty.

JENNY: I don't know. You're bleeding (*pointing to her mother's arm*).

DR. FISHMAN: Look at how they watch you. He says "Twenty," and she says "You're bleeding."

JENNY: Well, look at her arm.

DR. FISHMAN (*to Herb*): Did you see that? The way she says "You're bleeding," as though her mother were not competent enough to know that her own body is bleeding?

I am using every opportunity to magnify the youngsters' toxic enmeshment.

HERB: I swear to God. She doesn't even know when she's bleeding.

GREG: She never knows when she's hurt.

DR. FISHMAN (*to Herb*): And this has got to change. You see, they play this game. She says, "If I gain a few pounds," and they say, "Please gain a few pounds." And this has gone around for years already.

To end the session I intensify the message to the father that he must take control and challenge the mother to change.

HERB: It has gotten worse and she has gotten thinner.

DOROTHY: I want to stop it.

DR. FISHMAN: She says she wants to stop it, but don't believe it for a minute. These are nice kids.

DOROTHY: I want to stop it.

JENNY: No, you don't.

DOROTHY: Yes I *do*, I really do!

DR. FISHMAN (*to Herb*): You're the one who's got to change it. I think you just have to do it by fiat. You just have to take control.

By working with the children in this way I was working to free them. If the father acted as an umbrella, shielding the youngsters, then they could get to work on their own development. I did not feel at this point that they had had significant developmental lacunae.

Therapy with the Couple

Once the other forces destabilizing the system had been peeled away the couple became a true therapeutic entity, and we could now work on that unit. One week after the session with the children I had a session with Dorothy and Herb alone; its effects could be seen in a dramatic episode that followed. After this session Dorothy had another bout of electrolyte imbalance and was rushed to the hospital. When Herb went to see her he did not act guilty and sympathetic. On the contrary, he felt furious with his wife and threatened to leave. I believe that this couple had come away from their therapy session with a new template for handling severe problems: direct confrontation. Once his wife had directly confronted him, Herb felt that he could hit back when struck. He no longer owed anything, and so he could threaten to leave. Out of this dramatic antihomeostatic episode came the final movement toward health. Indeed, this was the last such episode on Dorothy's part of gorging herself on laxatives.

The session begins with the couple's reversion to their old pattern of gaslighting. I decide to call them on it.

DR. FISHMAN:	No, it's not. He just did it to you again. There goes the gaslight.
HERB:	What? "It's all in your mind?"
DR. FISHMAN:	Yes, by saying, "It's all in your mind."
DOROTHY:	But it isn't in my mind.
DR. FISHMAN (*to Dorothy*):	You see what you did? You accepted it.
DOROTHY:	I know. I know.
DR. FISHMAN:	Change him. The question is, can you be you? Can you be you—a full, robust person?
DOROTHY:	You know, unfortunately, that's what I basically was.
DR. FISHMAN:	Can you be a full person and have him love you?

In this family there was a fixed complementary pattern—Dorothy being sick and Herb responding—that stabilized the system. In the functional family, however, both the complementary (nurturing, reciprocal) behaviors and the symmetrical (competitive, challenging) behaviors need to be present. The goal of the session was to work with the couple until the missing pattern, symmetry, emerged. This session would end when Dorothy was able to challenge her husband and her husband was able to challenge back.

DOROTHY (*to Herb*):	You know, when I did this, I told you what I was doing. I made a conscious decision at that time to get thin like this. I knew I could do it. And I knew that that would be really a way of turning myself off from you. And I told you at the time. And you said, "You don't need it." And I said, "Yes, I do." I really had to. You never paid any attention to me. You really never did.
HERB:	Well, if you die, I can't pay attention to you either.
DOROTHY:	But you pay attention to me when I'm sick. You were so busy, so busy with your job and your house, and you never talked about us. There was always, "Did you get the cement block? Did you order the bricks? . . . It was the house, the house, the house. "Did you go to the antique course today?" So that I could learn more to be what you wanted me to be. And I couldn't function. Because I needed you and you were never really there. You were never really there—ever.
HERB:	Well, I guess that is my fault.
DOROTHY:	So I decided, who needs it. Rather than stay the way I was and go to somebody else, I told you what I was doing, I said I really wanted to keep this marriage, because I want the children and I want to be a good mother. And that's what I want more than needing somebody. But I think that I fight getting out of it, because I'm afraid there won't be anything there when I come out. And what do I do then? I mean, what happens if I come out of all this and get better and there's nothing there any more?

This is Dorothy's existential dilemma, her mid-life assessment of her situation. It took quite some courage for Dorothy to get better.

HERB:	Anybody that has gone through all this crap would have left you long ago (*he laughs*).

DOROTHY: But maybe there's nothing there anymore. Maybe you're going to stay, but maybe there won't be anything left of *us* any more. Of course you will stay. It's too convenient to leave. Who else is going to be as good a cook? And who else is going to iron all those shirts real nice, and make sure the collars are starched? You come home at 7:00, you go to sleep at 9:00. But I never tell you anything about it. You say, "Do you mind if I close my eyes?" No, I don't mind if you close your eyes. At one time I told you I was going to drink too much because then at least I would go to sleep. I couldn't even do that. Because that was doing something. I can only deprive myself.

DR. FISHMAN: I see Herb as very committed to this relationship.

DOROTHY: He really is.

DR. FISHMAN: Don't speak for him—because it's not fair. He needs to speak for himself. (*To Herb:*) I see you as very committed to Dorothy. But somehow Dorothy doesn't hear it. So what can you do to help? Do you feel committed to her?

HERB: Yes, very much so. I think she knows that. We wouldn't be here if. . . .

DR. FISHMAN: Herb, she doesn't know that. Because she just said she doesn't. Tell her.

HERB (*to Dorothy*): Why the hell do you think we're here? Why do you think I leave work every time to come here? Do you think it's because I want you to pour your soul out in front of the TV cameras? It would have been much easier to go and get a new wife. Dorothy, you know that I try to do everything for you that I can. Not everything, but I try to do what I think will make you comfortable.

The individuals in a system must be addressed as free agents who can dismantle or renew the system of which they are a part. In order to understand human systems we must speak to the issue of the freedom *not* to be a member of the system. At this point the couple is facing the fundamental issues of commitment and making choices. They have to recontract as free agents and the therapist must address them as two people who must be tapped as individuals in terms of commitment. At this moment I feel a little bit like a clergyman. I might as well be asking Herb, "Do you take this woman?" for I am asking this man if he is committed. That is an essential question in couples therapy.

DOROTHY: Do you know what I think?

HERB: What?

DOROTHY: I have said this before, too. I think you want to get me better because you have no idea of what is going to happen. You have forgotten what I am going to be like if I get better. And it's too comfortable for you. It is much easier to keep the wife and keep me from dying, or whatever. But have me because I'm used to you. I don't think you'd ever be able to break somebody else in. Because I don't think you would ever, at this point, ever be able to bamboozle what is young now. They're too smart. They really are.

A level of analysis is missing. While I have obtained a fairly honest, candid response, an expression of commitment from Herb, the system's inertia leads to redundantly seeing everything as the same. Dorothy sees her husband's movement as just one more step to hold her because he is afraid to branch out and get another wife. Of course, there is an element of truth in this. But part of the stagnation in this system is that new behavior is not recognized. He will have to fight more strongly to convey to her that he is committed.

HERB: Dorothy, you're trying to rationalize why you shouldn't get better.

DOROTHY: No, I am not.

DR. FISHMAN: Can you reassure Dorothy that you want a strong wife? That you want a wife who will be there for you? That you want a wife who's a real person, and not a skeleton?

HERB: Oh, I've tried to tell her that many times, but . . .

DR. FISHMAN: Well, tell her again now. Because I see you as competent. And I can't imagine a competent guy who would want a wife who is a waif, someone who's going to blow away. Or am I wrong?

HERB: No, you're right.

DR. FISHMAN: Then tell her. And make her hear you, because she doesn't hear you.

HERB: Dorothy, I don't want a wife who is going to blow away. Whatever blows her away—the wind, or the next plague that comes through.

DOROTHY: Okay. But will you want me the way I am going to come out of this? Are you really going to be happy with what comes out? Because I don't think you will be. And that's why I am not convinced.

If therapy with ossified, rigid systems such as this one is to be effective, there must be a moment like this, orchestrated by the therapist. The couple must be brought to a rewriting of the fundamental rules of the relationship and a revising of their contract. This is not a charade. The therapy has permitted strangers to enter into a new way of bonding, and these two people have revised the nature of their tie. At this moment they are individuals in the process of recontracting. If the process is real, the individuals will show honest reluctance, and the reluctance will indicate that it is not a guaranteed, sure thing.

Another metaphor suggested here is that of birth, of something new emerging. When systems therapy hits a crossroad like this the participants will begin talking about transformation and the birth of new identities. The process makes clear that choices will have to be made, because the transformation of the participants cannot be totally anticipated and requires a new contract.

DOROTHY: And I think I need more of an investment of you. I really do.

HERB: I give you sympathy when I—when I—correct you—or whatever I'm supposed to be doing.

DOROTHY: But I'm not a child. I don't correct you. Why would you correct me? You are you, why would I correct you?

HERB: Well, I used the wrong word.

A key moment of misapprehension has been revealed. The participants have entered into a kind of parent-to-child model which is inappropriate to a marriage. In the fixed system of this family Dorothy is the child: she is one-down. The goal of the therapy is for the system to be sufficiently flexible so that they can mother and father each other as well as challenge.

HERB: If you want to call it criticism. Two people can't live together, I don't think, without having something critical to say about one another every now and then.

DOROTHY: I don't mind if it is on a personal level, between us. Just don't criticize me in front of the kids. Just don't do that. It is going to be hard. And I don't think you can undo it now. The pattern has been so established.

DR. FISHMAN: You can undo it if you stop.

This is an important notion about family history. This history is to some extent recursively connected to the present. On the basis of the present context, each person will screen history differently and select different things as germane.

DOROTHY:	All right, you can stop it—you can stop it. But what's there is there. Now, somehow, I've got to get back Gregory's respect.
DR. FISHMAN:	You'll do that. But you didn't get his (*indicating Herb*).
HERB:	You got mine, Dorothy. I have respect for you.
DOROTHY:	If you did, you wouldn't do that.
HERB:	No. If I didn't, I wouldn't do it. Why would I want to see you make a fool out of yourself when you're doing something irrational?
DR. FISHMAN:	Dorothy, Herb didn't agree.
HERB:	No. I agree. I would like you to get your strong personality back, and be independent, and have Gregory respect you, and everybody else in the world respect you.
DOROTHY:	I can't do that unless I have your help. You, Herb, have to express some respect for me.

In terms of the multi-faceted self and of reality confirmed by significant others Dorothy cannot be strong and respect herself unless she has a context that respects her.

HERB:	I will stop.
DOROTHY:	In front of the children—that's the big thing. Not just remain neutral, because you're big at remaining neutral on everything.
HERB:	Well, I will step in and stick up for you when I think you're right. When I think you're wrong, I'll ignore it.
DOROTHY:	Every once in a while I may have a good idea. What's wrong with saying, "Your mother had a great idea"? My great idea this year consisted of "Let's go to Bear World." That was my big, good idea.
HERB:	It rained.
DOROTHY:	I mean—I really come up with some terrific ones.

The couple was revealing the skewed pattern in which they lived, a pattern in which he was always up and she was always down. Dorothy was disclosing the areas where she was devalued—specifically, her intellectual prowess. With the therapist's support she remembered how Herb always picked up on her most silly and infantile ideas, selectively shutting out her moments of substantial and creative thought. Throughout this session I chiseled away, working discretely on the process of identifying the moments when Dorothy was being gaslighted and when she was contributing to putting herself down. This is a process that cannot be rushed; one must watch for moments of entrapment and identify them right then and there.

One of the most fortunate developments in in-depth family therapy is that it is possible, through extreme disruption of fundamental homeostatic maintainers, to release people not only to change but to change their reason for changing. One such sequence takes place in the next segment. Dorothy recognizes that she will change, but not for her children's sake or even for her husband's sake. The change will be strictly for herself. With this kind of development one realizes that the disruption of the homeostatic maintainer has been complete. This couple is really to the point of reformulating and renegotiating the contract. The gaslighting has been dismantled completely, and what emerges is two individuals, each contemplating a relationship with the other. At this point they are no longer systematized.

The therapist is keenly aware when the system has been rendered asystemic and does not rush to allow the couple to regain security and to resystematize, to become a unit again. If that happens the session is likely to end with the relationship in a continuing dilemma. I guarantee nothing and make it quite clear that I am not interested in having them settle down. She finishes and he finishes, and I deliberately try to control the scenario so that when they exit they are an unresolved chord.

Previously, in order to preserve the system, this couple had to accommodate. What I try to do is make the accommodation itself be at stake. I am not about to try to end this session on a happy note. My emphasis is on exiting very fast. It is the nature of the play that is at stake, and these two people do not even know if they want to be in this play together. The goal of good therapy should be to increase the family members' recognition of the freedom they have to enter or leave the play. This amounts to resisting a homeostatic retrieval. If the couple wants to go back and latch onto another way of being a unit, the therapist should block it. The idea is to disengage them as parts of a system and leave them as people who have to negotiate a new way of integrating.

DR. FISHMAN: Now you're putting yourself down. You are inviting your husband to disrespect you.

DOROTHY: Why do I do that?

DR. FISHMAN: I don't know why. After you are better you can find out why.

DOROTHY: But I need to stop that.

DR. FISHMAN: Of course you do. You're inviting him to disrespect you.

HERB: And you do the same thing with the kids.

DR. FISHMAN: You take great care of this family. You are a very productive person. The question is, will your husband take you, not only in sickness . . .

HERB: But in health. I will take you well and in health this time.

DOROTHY: Okay. But up until now I've been afraid to take the chance. I don't want to risk that. Do you want to know why I don't want to risk that?

(Herb laughs.)

DR. FISHMAN: He's daring you. He is saying that you are not really going to change.

DOROTHY: He said, "I've seen it before."

DR. FISHMAN: I think you are going to change.

HERB: Well, I'm waiting.

DOROTHY: Do you know what I really want to say to you? I am going to change. Whether you wind up in the picture or not.

HERB: Well, that is what I like to hear.

DOROTHY: I am not quite ready to do that. I can't really bring myself to that thinking. But right now that is what I want to do.

DR. FISHMAN: You know you need to.

Dorothy is now able to really challenge her husband and he is able to challenge her back. This is the emergence of a new pattern. Now my aim is to increase the intensity, to push it above the homeostatic threshold.

DOROTHY: I can't support myself and the kids, not the way those children are used to being supported. I can't ever provide a life style for them like that, so the thought really panics me. But I have to say to you that if I come out of this, and I am okay through it all physically, my personality will be what it is. And if you don't like it, and it really bothers you enough to leave, then I will make my way, no matter what.

HERB: If your personality changes to where you are—where you can't hang in there anymore, then I guess we do leave, or whatever. But I don't think that is going to happen.

DOROTHY: Okay. I just keep remembering that in 1976, when I made that attempt, and I was quite well on my way—I weighed 115 pounds then—it wasn't worth it. I remember thinking, this isn't working. Nothing changed. I kept promising myself that you and I would change, but it didn't get any better. And I said, forget it. I am better off the way I was.

What is evident in Dorothy's presentation is the significance of the history of a system in evolution, the developmental aspects of a family system. Dorothy is making references to the point in the history of their relationship when she decided to get thinner and thinner. And in part this decision illustrates the darker side of human nature; we realize that part of the homeostatic arrangement is what used to be called, in theological circles, vindictiveness. Somehow Dorothy decided to rob her husband of a wife. At the same time she was robbing herself of a healthy life and full personality.

HERB: You know, Dorothy, just because someone has a disagreement, or an argument—everybody has arguments.

DOROTHY: They are not arguments. It is constant ignoring. Do you realize now that I am getting more attention from you than I have ever gotten in eighteen years?

HERB: I am very concerned about it.

DOROTHY: I am in my glory. I am getting all this attention and all I had to do is get sick for it.

HERB: But that is a child's way of thinking. That is what I keep saying. Or what he has told us.

DOROTHY: I feel stronger now and I can confront you and say that I don't want to be ignored any more.

HERB: If life is that bad, go out and leave me, or something. But you don't punish yourself by getting sick.

DOROTHY: I don't know why that motherhood thing was so important to me. It was so important that I be the good woman and keep the family together. I just at that time could not face the thought that I needed you, and you were not there. And maybe I would find someone else.

Seldom do we find such clear evidence of this darker side of human nature, a side where people choose to employ an indomitable will in expressing vindictiveness toward another person. When Dorothy recalled those past events we saw an attempt to abandon killing herself, an attempt to get well and gain weight. But this attempt ceased when she discovered that the world was not going to fall at her feet. Her husband did not rave about the fact that she was holding weight and getting well. Rather, her husband continued to be unavailable to her. As a result Dorothy resorted to vindictiveness and returned to her anorexia. This is a more common pattern among anorexics than might be supposed. It is clear that in starving themselves, these people are attacking others.

In contrast to her failed attempt at change, the renewed effort Dorothy described in the last sequence was far more positive and less dependent on the response of others. She was clearly saying, "I am going to change whether you like it or not." By taking this stand she was forcing Herb to change as well and to help maintain and acknowledge her own change. This time she was saying, "I can do without the applause; I'll applaud myself, thank you"—quite an emancipating step.

Her husband's response to this new emancipation was mixed. Herb's language reflected the kind of dryness that had helped form his wife's emotional desert. It lacked emotional intensity. But there were glimpses of the positive. Though somewhat reluctantly, he did convey to Dorothy his acceptance of the notion that they would end the relationship if part of her getting well would be an insistence on leaving. Later this thought was amplified in a way I liked better: of his wife's anorexia Herb said, "Go out and leave me, or something. But you don't punish yourself by getting sick." This declaration showed his commitment to her well-being. I believe it was Elizabeth Kubler Ross who coined the phrase "heroic love." Within Dorothy's husband there is a capacity for extraordinary love. He is signaling that he would rather keep the tie with her, but he has the courage to lose her if it means she will live. It is significant that this moment follows his wife's explanation of how her anorexia is a mechanism of revenge, a self-punishment designed also to punish him. In response the husband now revises the contract and says, "I'd rather you go free than punish yourself." In this expression of heroic love, he transcends his own needs and takes the first step toward reforming the unequal bond he has had with his wife.

This point would not have been reached in the therapy if the other, intrusive parts of the system had not been removed. The intrusion of the parental and child subsystems would have interfered with generating the necessary intensity. It is this intensity that brings the key issues to the surface. In the sequence that follows the issues are guilt and blame.

DR. FISHMAN: See, Herb, what she is telling you, in a sense, is that it is all
                 your fault. That you ignore her.

> HERB: Yeah, well, I am getting that.
>
> DR. FISHMAN: The thing is, she lets you ignore her. She could wake you at 9:00. She could meet you in town. She could insist that you go away for a weekend.

The point of therapy here is to not allow the husband to be burdened with the sins of the total process. This sequence also has a serendipitous by-product. By utilizing this tool of guilt-leveling we can bring out any injustices undealt with, any grievances not settled, any accounts not yet paid.

The accumulated sins of the marriage are all revealed. The couple is righting a wrong, reordering a skewed relationship to bring it back to parity. This sequence contains a kind of ultimate purging which must be experienced before the relationship can right itself and make possible a fresh start.

In the sequence that follows I continue to further the process by escalating the intensity, supporting the husband in order to draw Dorothy out and give her something to push against.

> DR. FISHMAN: All right. She could take you out to dinner. She could get you to take her out to dinner. She could have parties and she doesn't. And I don't know why she doesn't.
>
> HERB: Why aren't you more aggressive in those areas?
>
> DOROTHY: I was—and you told me I was disgusting—to go away from you. Listen, you have a very short memory. I think about it. And don't say things like that. Don't put me through this, okay?
>
> HERB: Dorothy, going out to dinner, meeting me in town, those things I have asked you if you wanted to do.
>
> DOROTHY: Why? So you can get drunk and fall asleep?
>
> HERB: Oh, come on. We go away. Maybe we don't go away enough, because we can't afford it.
>
> DOROTHY: I have gone away with you, okay. I can name you times—years—where you never went to bed with me. If I ask you, I am disgusting. [You say,] "Go away from me."
>
> HERB: Oh, come on. We have a disagreement about something and you let it build up in your head.
>
> DOROTHY: You forget. You get drunk and you say those things. You have a very short memory.

The ability to remember is important. The fact is that a system has a history, and in order to produce lasting change that is coherent with the family's experience we must talk about the significance of damage and of repairing damage. As the system is transformed the participants realize that they can enter into new complementarity. "We don't have to remain stuck back there," they say, "because we have settled some of the damage; it has been repaired."

There is a school of thought that new patterns of complementarity can be structured without having a process of renewal and amnesis and repair of damage. In my view, when the sense of injury among the participants runs deep it is extremely important to have a meticulous, detailed revision of areas in which damage has been felt. This process entails the retrieval of memories and injury and the offering of an opportunity to attack the person responsible for past hurts. In addition, there must be an opportunity for the one who did the hurting to feel that the sins have been expiated. It is from this kind of dialogue that a new accountability arises that can help further the process of revising the couple's contract and structuring a new complementarity.

This couple's dialogue involved a discrete review of specific injuries and a settling of old accounts. The wife got back at her husband, the husband found out that he had to ask for forgiveness, and the wife decided to grant it. This entire process followed from carefully maneuvering the couple into a situation where they could discover two things: that the wife could attack her husband, and that the husband can stand being attacked.

The wife in this system remained caught between wanting to stay in the family, with a husband who came to her only when she was sick, and living in a psychosomatic system where everything was supposed to be perfect. This extreme split had consequences: recall that the immediate outcome of this exercise in reviewing and repairing a list of discrete abuses to the self was that the wife had another anorexic crisis. This time, however, the husband felt he owed her nothing and so could threaten to leave. What had transpired up to this point allowed this man to feel that he had answered for the cumulative grievances in the relationship and that now they must go on to something new.

HERB: But isn't part of life forgiving and forgetting, and going on?

DOROTHY: Yes, but I can't. I told you that meant a lot to me. I told you—you kick me out once too often—and that was it. And you did. I told you, "You will never do that to me again, ever." Never, never again. Now you forget all these things. But I don't forget them. Because they were very, very painful, really painful. It is only now that I can even talk about it. You wonder why I think there is something wrong with me—I think you have given me every reason

	to think that there is something wrong with me. My whole way was not the way a lovely woman and a mother should behave.
DR. FISHMAN:	What about from now on; what do you want?
HERB:	What I said before—come out of this thing and whatever your personality is . . .
DOROTHY:	I don't think you could handle me. Honest to goodness—I don't think you could.
HERB:	If I can't, I can't.
DOROTHY:	But are you going to make me feel like some sort of an inferior creep—like a streetwalker? Are you going to make me feel common? I don't want to be common, because I'm not really.
HERB:	I never said you were.
DOROTHY:	I don't believe you. I don't believe you.
DR. FISHMAN:	See, Dorothy thinks you are weak. She thinks you are very weak. The only way she can support you as a husband is by being weaker. And I don't think you are weak. I think you can take having a strong wife. You will be more alive than you have ever been.
HERB:	I think I can too.
DR. FISHMAN:	You better tell her that. I think you will be ten times more alive than you were a year ago, when you have a strong wife.
HERB:	Dorothy, I want you to come out of this and be a strong personality—or whatever it takes.
DOROTHY:	If you are willing to take the chance.
HERB:	I'll take the chance. Is it a deal?
DR. FISHMAN:	Shake on it.
DOROTHY:	Hey, I can't take the humiliation again, you know that.
HERB:	There will be no humiliation.
DOROTHY:	You know I can't face that.
HERB:	There will be no humiliation. Shake.
DOROTHY (*shaking his hand*):	I will have to think whether it is worth it.
DR. FISHMAN:	It is worth it. The fact is you don't really have a choice. Because if you don't do it, you'll die—either physically or emotionally.

(I get up, put on my jacket, and walk out of the room.)

By the end of the session a symmetrical pattern has emerged. Dorothy challenges her husband, "I don't think it's worth it. I want to come out of this and be a strong person or whatever it takes," and her husband responds, "I want you to come out of this and become a strong personality." The therapist monitors the emergence of corrective patterns. This is a system that has been stuck in a complementary sequence and where Dorothy has always been one down. At the end of this session there was a new pattern emerging. They could both be symmetrical. For both spouses to challenge each other was an indication to the therapist that the session had achieved its goal.

Herb had emotionally hit his wife once too often and Dorothy had not had an opportunity to give him the detailed, formidable thrashing that he deserved. When she finally did, it was extremely liberating for this man. That was why later, when she tried a desperate move—gorging herself with laxatives, leading to coma and hospitalization—she came to and found him freed. What she saw was an annoyed man who could in fact actually leave her because he had no debts. One only stays around if one has debts.

About three weeks after the coma episode Dorothy and Herb came to me with another problem: their lack of a sexual life together. I was not surprised by this complaint, for their lack of sexual intimacy was evident from the distance between the two. Although I am not a sex therapist, I decided that rather than referring them to a specialist, who would create another uncertainty in this system, I would first try my own home-grown approach at solutions. I suggested that they begin by buying the book *The Joy of Sex* and perusing it as a manual. Considering Dorothy's training as a "proper girl," the mere act of buying this type of book was one more opportunity to challenge her tendency to avoid conflict and her compulsive good-girlness. I also suggested that they see some X-rated movies. In the following weeks they went through the book and saw some movies, and they reported that their sex life had improved. In actuality I think the book and movies had very little to do with it. I attribute the amelioration of the sexual problem to the same process that made them bring it up in the first place: if they saw it as a difficulty, then clearly they were ready for more intimacy and had come to realize that sexual intimacy was important to them. They were now a couple. Dorothy was a wife, not just a daughter to her parents, and Herb was now an active husband. As a couple they could now address their problem and have a conjugal relationship rather than remaining two adolescents living around the block from their parents.

A few months later, following the termination of their therapy, Dorothy called me to say she had another problem. "My parents are fighting like cats and dogs," she reported, "since I stopped being available and spending so much time there." I offered my services, but Dorothy said that she had decided her parents were having "growing pains" and that they would work it out themselves.

As mentioned earlier, in working with adolescents the key pivotal conflict involves in many ways the parental couple. Once the couple has been transformed, by being seen in therapy alone as a couple as well as with the rest of the family, new patterns will emerge that will affect the children. Triangulation and conflicts can be resolved in the presence of the children, and conflicts can be resolved between the children in the presence of the parents without the parents intervening. Once this stage is accomplished then one has a sense that the therapeutic goals have been reached.

A consistent metaphor used in this book is that of the adolescents being in orbit around the adult dyad, whether this consists of a mother and father whose marriage is intact, a divorced couple still connected, or any other adult parental figures. The parental subsystem for many families continues to be the nucleus around which the children orbit. It is for this reason that it is so essential to end therapy only when that system is stabilized and functioning well according to the principles enumerated in this chapter. If we imagine a solar system where the nucleus is unstable, unpredictable, and busy tearing itself apart, we can easily conjecture the catastrophic effects on the outlying planets. As it goes on the astronomical realm, so it goes on the level of individual families. And that is why as family therapists we must pay such close attention to the couple as the center of the family system.

11

Follow-up

Oने OF the key assumptions made in this book is that the therapist works not only toward the amelioration of the family's presenting
symptom but also toward the stabilization and maintenance of new structures within the system. Follow-up sessions conducted at set intervals or in
response to calls for help form an essential part of the overall therapy. This
book cannot provide extensive follow-up material for each of the cases
presented, but it can take a look at the follow-up done with one family and
analyze its implications.

The family I chose to illustrate the follow-up approach and technique
is the family introduced in the previous chapter on couples therapy. The
therapy had succeeded in assisting the couple to work through their history, redress grievances, and begin the difficult process of forgiveness and
a renegotiation of their contract together. During the course of therapy
with Dorothy and Herb, Dorothy had a disastrous fight with her father,
took a huge number of laxatives, and went into a coma. When her husband
came to see her in the hospital there occurred a dramatic confrontation:
Herb made it clear that he and Dorothy should part if that was what it
would take to keep her well. After this confrontation Dorothy did stay well
and she has not to date abused laxatives. The exploration of the follow-up

with this couple concerns itself with the patterns of effective change and their maintenance.

I believe the single most important concept for follow-up is Gregory Bateson's dormitive principle (see Keeney 1983). This notion refers to the intellectual error of confusing the name of the problem with the context that maintains the problem. In this case the name of the problem is the children's depression and the mother's severe anorexia. The context that maintains the problem is the dysfunctional system that was described and treated in the previous chapter. Thus the follow-up should address the status of the individual problem and, just as important, it should evaluate the context and changes in the context.

ONE-YEAR FOLLOW-UP

One year following therapy I phoned and asked Dorothy, "Do you remember me?" She answered, "Yes, we were just speaking of you last week." Concerned, I inquired further. Dorothy replied, "There was a trip to Florida advertised on the TV, and I said to myself, thinking about you, "You know, we should have the driveway paved, but what the heck, it's better if Herb and I go on a vacation." During this conversation I asked Dorothy what she thought was keeping her well. First, she said that she would never become ill again because her children had done so beautifully after she got better. (Greg had just spent the summer in Europe with his team, and Jenny was on the school newspaper and doing very well.) Then she said, "The second thing I learned was to stay out of my parents' marriage."

TWO-YEAR FOLLOW-UP

Two years and three months after the cessation of therapy I invited the family back for a follow-up interview. I framed this event as a research tool and not as a therapeutic session. Dorothy, Herb, and Jenny arrived for the interview. Greg was too busy with his friends and school.

EVALUATING THE SYSTEM

To assess process I first had this family undergo an interactional diagnostic family task, the family task described in the book *Psychosomatic Families* (Minuchin, Rosman, and Baker 1978). I then scored the instrument impressionistically, using my clinical judgment, in an attempt to ascertain whether the family still manifested the patterns of a psychosomatic family: conflict avoidance, diffusion of conflict, rigidity, enmeshment, and overprotectiveness. While observing this task I prepared my questions for the second part of the follow-up interview.

The second part involved seeing the family together and also as subsystems. I saw the individuals in different subsystems because I believed that it would violate boundaries to ask the couple about their marriage in the presence of the daughter. Similarly, Dorothy's anorexia was her own business. I first saw Dorothy, Herb, and Jenny (the son was too busy to attend). I observed the atmosphere in the room: did they seem to feel comfortable together? How was the daughter doing? Was she still glued to the home, caring for her mother? Did she feel free to go off and attend to her own needs? What about the son? Was he still at home because the system needed him there to stabilize the parents' relationship? Was he at home simply for convenience? I already believed, on the basis of the family task, that there was no longer the diffusion of conflict. But I could not be certain because this was an informational interview.

Once I had ascertained that things seemed to be in good shape, I was interested to know what the family members had done differently so that this new, happier status quo was maintained. Was there a new organization that accompanied the newfound happiness?

I then saw just the couple. I wanted to know how they felt about their relationship. Were they still locked into a dysfunctional struggle, either symmetrical or complementary? I wanted their assessment regarding how the children and the grandparents were doing. Again, I wanted to know what had changed in the family structure.

The third part of this interview involved seeing Dorothy alone. In this setting I asked about her anorexia. I again wanted to know what she thought had changed in the system that rendered everyone happier.

Transformation and Growth

The systems therapist must examine not only whether the system is being transformed in terms of dysfunctional patterns but also the extent and nature of the transformation. Is there sufficient transformation so that the adolescents are free to expand into other contexts that augment development? Are there developmental lacunae? In terms of our follow-up family have the two children fallen developmentally behind their peers because they had spent so many years taking care of their mother? After all, when their friends were at the mall or playing sports, they were sitting at home observing their mother's every move, fearing she might at any given moment go into another coma. At the cessation of therapy it is the therapist's responsibility to make sure that the children are at least on the road to achieving developmental maturation.

In our follow-up session the fact that the son, Greg, did not attend seemed to me good news. It suggested that he was more appropriately attached to the extrafamilial context and not, as he had been during the therapy, tethered to the home and the family. Of course I needed more information to complete the picture. For all I knew, Greg might have disengaged from the context only to become involved in the drug culture. My goal in the following sequence was to ascertain to what extent Greg had disengaged.

HERB:	Greg is out of high school and in college. Jenny's a sophomore. Dorothy's got her head screwed on straight.
JENNY:	Mom has gotten into personal fitness.

We see an old pattern that never really changed. Herb snipes at Dorothy and Jenny supports her.

DOROTHY:	I have to rechannel my energy somewhere. I'm using the same amount of energy towards doing something constructive.
DR. FISHMAN:	Very good. Sounds great. Now, where is Greg going to college?
HERB:	He's going to the state college nearby, so that's why he's still home.
DR. FISHMAN:	So he's still living at home.
HERB:	Yes.
DR. FISHMAN:	And how is that?
HERB:	He's all right . . .
DOROTHY:	Someday he'll move out of the bedroom.
HERB (*laughing*):	He's all right—he just doesn't want to leave his happy home.
DR. FISHMAN:	What do you think that's all about?
DOROTHY:	Comfort. He keeps saying, "I can get a good meal at home, why should I go eat school food?" You know—he has his own bed and his own phone and a car, and he can come in any time at night. He's got a place to live. Except I think a lot of it is immaturity, too. I think that if he lived away from home he would have to be on his own and make new friends and be in a situation where he was unfamiliar with the surroundings. And it's very difficult to push him out and say you have to be there. Hopefully, he will do it eventually.

HERB:	He's got to because he can only go there for two years.
DOROTHY:	After that he's got to go somewhere else.
DR. FISHMAN:	Does he have friends?
DOROTHY:	He has a lot of friends.
DR. FISHMAN:	Girlfriend?
JENNY:	No.
HERB:	Not yet.
JENNY:	Girls call. He's got girl *friends*, as in . . .
DOROTHY:	I don't think he has, like, a girlfriend.

The fact that Greg has a lot of friends is very important. If he had a girlfriend it would signify a different level of disengagement, a closer step toward separation. It concerns me that he does not, and I wonder whether there is something that we could have done in the therapy to have made him more autonomous and disengaged.

DR. FISHMAN (*to Jenny*):	Do you two fight a lot?
JENNY:	We don't talk. I mean, he has his friends, who are not my friends, and the only time we talk is when he's yelling at me because of the car or something like that. I mean, we talk, say hi and stuff, and sometimes we go to the same parties and will be at the same place, you know, but we don't associate together.

The family did not undergo a remarkable transformation, but it did modify itself to accommodate Greg's moratorium. Obviously, they wanted him to get out, but they accommodated somewhat to his need for an intermediate step. The overall direction, however, had been set, and the mother, father, and sister were aware that Greg was hanging on a bit long.

The parents' response did not indicate a system that needed the son to stay home as a homeostatic maintainer. One could sense flexibility and accommodation, but the main goal—that he would have to leave—was not lost. In fact, this family had established guidelines for when Greg would move out, guidelines that suggest that the system was ready to release him yet willing to accommodate a bit longer because there were problems involving his readiness. This was realistic. After all, this system was stuck for quite a while, and its history must have taken a toll in the flight capacities of the adolescent.

In retrospect I think it would have been beneficial to have done, in the initial sessions, more work with the young man himself to address these developmental lacunae. The danger is, of course, that one will create a therapy that becomes "terminally interminable." I prefer a model of therapy in which the therapist moves in, makes a change, and leaves the door open the way general practitioners do.

Has the Oldest Adolescent Left Home?

Figuratively speaking, there was another adolescent living in this family: the mother. And she, too, underwent considerable development and liberation. There was good evidence of the mother's ability to disengage from her own parents and escape a powerful pattern of enmeshment. We must ask, however, if there were now clear methods for boundary making. Boundaries can be effected through brief therapy, a therapy directed at the salient issues—the joints in the system. The relationship between Dorothy and her parents was clearly an infected joint. Yet apparently the change did not necessitate a complete break. The firm upholding of boundaries between Dorothy and her parents undoubtedly created some friction and some crises, but these did not mean that she had ejected these people from her life. Instead, what occurred was a reorganization of boundaries that allowed Dorothy to remain in contact with her mother and father, but in a relationship with rules for controlling intrusiveness.

Boundary reorganization is not simply an issue of dependence versus independence, as self-actualization theory or psychoanalytic development theory would have us believe. It is more a matter of shifting dependencies into interdependencies, but with new rules that permit space for growth in all participants. The way in which Dorothy and her husband disengaged from her parents also served as a model for their two children. My hope was that the children would learn that leaving home is not running away—it is walking away. One of Dorothy's difficulties was that *her* mother had never successfully negotiated Dorothy's departure from home. In fact, Dorothy's grandmother had been very much involved during Dorothy's mother's entire married life in the personal affairs of their family.

A firm boundary is one that is built specifically to resist the parents' efforts at triangulating their daughter into their unresolved marital conflict.

DOROTHY: I just refused outright to discuss anything with their marriage at all. If it would come up, I would leave the room or say, "I'm not going to talk about that—that's out." And then when I refused to talk about it, they started talking to one another. They really did get back together again. But

it took a long time, didn't it? It took about a year before
they got back together again. But then they took a trip
together and I found a senior citizens group for my
mother to belong to and then she got a circle of friends.
And I moved them out of my life, but I can't say that I
didn't manipulate it, because I really did, I mean I kind of
had to channel things. I got my father a job as a maître d'.

DR. FISHMAN: It's good to do a little therapy.

DOROTHY: I wouldn't say that it was therapy; what I did was, I tried
to get them out of my life without hurting their feelings.

Notice that Dorothy, who said she had cut these people out of her life,
was still responsibly connected to them. The transformations that had to
occur did not really call for a total severance of ties. It was not an amputa-
tion, but a shifting of relationships in certain key areas. Furthermore,
Dorothy's disengagement was followed by a re-engagement on another
level. Only to the extent that she became a responsible grown daughter
could she get her parents out of her life and successfully disengage.

It is clear that the therapy changed this woman to the extent that she
could now engineer the establishment of new boundaries between herself
and her family of origin. Before therapy she would continually get enmeshed in the private details and difficulties of her parents' marriage, a
situation that would draw her in and incapacitate her. In the follow-up
session she talked of controlling first the external intrusion—how often
they visited and called. She then got to more difficult ground—the psycho-
somatically dangerous areas that might have entailed her parents splitting,
being angry with each other, and leaving her. She was able to enter this
risky interpersonal domain because she had essentially freed herself from
her family of origin.

DR. FISHMAN: Okay. And how are they doing now?

DOROTHY: They're fine together. I wouldn't say that things are rosy,
but they're fine together. They're as good as I've ever seen
them. And that's great, because they like a certain amount
of hassle like that.

*This is an extraordinary development. Dorothy, upon re-
alizing that it was her parents' way to have a "certain
amount of hassle," knew that she could exit without trying to fix it.*

Has Herb Changed as a Husband and Father?

At one point in the follow-up Jenny mentioned that her father had changed in a very significant way: he was no longer upset when Dorothy went out to work, and in fact he supported it. Prior to therapy Herb was extremely resistant to the idea that Dorothy might want to work and establish an independent context of her own. This change was significant because it allowed Dorothy access to a different context that confirmed her as an individual and because it allowed her to feel much better about herself without the worry that she was somehow upsetting her husband.

HERB:	Can you tell if I've changed?
DR. FISHMAN:	Over the last twenty minutes?
DOROTHY (*to Herb*):	I think that's the biggest thing that I've noticed—that you're more tolerant and you spend more time with me.
HERB:	Well, I can't disagree, but if it's a change, I haven't noticed. I don't say I spend more time now than I did before. I think we do things more together because the kids are older and they're not around. Like we go out to dinner more together.

Obviously, the therapy had left lasting changes. Although he did not perceive it as a permanent change in his personality, both his wife and daughter attested to the fact that Herb had become more considerate. This recognition was unusual because not everybody accepts the reality of change easily. And indeed, the couple's interactions showed him to be more considerate—in the way he looked at Dorothy, listened to what she had to say, and he carefully chose his words. This dramatic change was a direct response to the intensity of the work done in therapy, the result of his wife's strong prodding and insistence. That Herb failed to acknowledge the change is not significant. It is enough that those around him saw him differently.

The Marriage

The change in this couple's marriage was extraordinary. The husband was clearly more available, they were more of a couple, and there was a sense of playfulness between them. The amnesia for the earlier difficulties was also impressive. We can account for this with the assumption that history is based on the present context. What people look for in the past is based on the parameters and characteristics of the present, and at present this couple was a happy, solid unit.

Not that all was perfect, of course. Herb still tended not to perceive his wife's power. Dorothy, however, was now ready to defend her own interests and was no longer a passive actor deferring to her husband. In addition, Herb had removed himself from the lifelong mission of trying to make his wife eat.

We should also take notice here of a different emotional tone in the couple's interaction. In the past, during therapy, Herb never permitted himself to be playful or to present himself in a "one-down" position. Now, not only was there playfulness, but he even allowed himself to be the buffoon. He came into the session with his galoshes on the wrong feet and allowed himself to be the butt of a playful joke.

So the follow-up session revealed that the therapy had in fact brought about important changes. There was now a respected boundary between the couple. Herb was no longer unhappy that his wife worked, and Dorothy had been given the space to develop herself. Furthermore, in terms of the system's rigidity, Herb was much more tolerant. In the past there had been difficulty because Herb felt that he had married beneath him and was always trying to raise his wife socially. In response, Dorothy would feel deeply rejected and act as if she were always walking on eggshells in her attempts to please her husband. In the sequence that follows, the family discusses the nature of the changes that have occurred.

DR. FISHMAN: What do you think changed, such that things got better? I'm going to ask each of you. Jenny, what do you think?

JENNY: In our family? What changed? Um—I think all the change happened to Mom, I guess. She's a lot less—um . . .

DOROTHY: You can say it.

JENNY: I know, I'm trying to think. Like, I'm not worried, because I mean she's fine now—now that she has a job and is really happy and everything. And when it comes to— she's not like, "Oh, you *have* to sit down and eat dinner." Sometimes she makes me go to bed but usually she's more like, "You want to eat at school, eat at school; you want to eat at home, eat at home." She's more relaxed. She's more confident, I think. He seems more relaxed, too. Most of the change has been in Mom. She's a lot more relaxed and it makes me feel good, *so I can go away without thinking,* "Oh, my God, I'm going to come home and see her curled up on the couch and in pain." I'm not worried about her any more.

Will the Kids Be Able to Leave Home?

Jenny's statement that she could leave home without fear of dire consequences may indeed have been the most important result of the entire therapy. Transformation of the system, Dorothy's freedom from her parents (as well as her parents from her), the creation of a boundary between the kids and their parents, and, finally, the spouses' reunion as a married couple resulted in growing space for this girl. She was still close to her parents, but she was not tethered to them. Her ability to grow was no longer being hindered by her intense ties to her sick mother.

When I asked Jenny what had changed in the family, Jenny went immediately to the heart of the issue: "I can leave now because my mother is fine." She pointedly brought out that she no longer had to be "on duty" as a watcher over her mother. In addition, both Jenny and her brother were doing very well in school and in their social development.

In the following segment Jenny had left the room and I concentrated on checking the state of the marriage relationship.

Checking the Marital Dyad

DR. FISHMAN: I want to ask you some questions about your marriage.

HERB: Go ahead.

DR. FISHMAN: What has changed, if anything, in your marriage? (*Pause.*) You might want to talk together about it.

HERB: Basically, I think that what's happened is that Dorothy's gotten rid of her mother and father—out of the house and out of our lives—and she's had more time to do things with the family, such as the kids or even myself. Plus her own self, which is more important than the three of us. Such as meeting friends, going out to lunch—you know—going to these different meetings that you have, and teaching the aerobics. Once she got her mother and father out of our lives the whole thing changed. When we first started here, we started with the premise that Dorothy's mother and father were mostly the problem.

Dorothy's changed relationship with her parents was a decisive turning point in the transformation of this couple's marriage. Dorothy began by blocking her parents' intrusion in her life. She then widened her own context, finding new relationships and creating a circle of friends. Applying these same lessons to her parents, she was also able to help them broaden their contexts. It is interesting that she worked avidly and intelligently at this transformation of both her and her parents' lives and that the combination proved so strong. It may have been that these patterns of enmeshment could not yield to boundary setting alone, but also required a careful assembly of alternate people and places for the intruding parties to focus on. In a sense, what Dorothy did was remain engaged with her parents enough to organize a satisfactory distance between them and herself.

Crisis: A Dangerous Opportunity

The system had changed during a point of crisis. Notice, however, that it was not just Dorothy's realization but also the effect of the crisis on the marriage that had propelled change.

HERB: And I think that was the culmination of it all. Then Dorothy finally realized at that time that she had to kick the monkey off her back or . . .

DR. FISHMAN: Did you really?

DOROTHY: Oh, absolutely. I thought, I'm going to kill myself, I'm going to die, or I'm going to get better right now, but it can't go on—it couldn't go on like that. I was filled with so much hatred. I can't even explain to you. I would be driving in a car and there would be this uncontrollable rage—all at once. I was going to go out of my mind—I mean I really was angry. And all my energy was being used up in this hatred and anger. I didn't have time for him. I didn't have time to even care for myself.

HERB: You didn't have time for anything. Not only me, you didn't have time for friends outside, the immediate family—what have you.

DR. FISHMAN: In terms of the two of you, what has changed now that your folks are off the scene?

DOROTHY: We do more things together. We go away a lot more together, don't you think?

HERB: Oh, yeah. We go out and we're together, and we've had to do things together. I mean, there's only the two of us and either you get along or you don't, and I think we've always gotten along fairly well without all these outside influences.

DOROTHY: I don't think we ever had anything basically wrong with the marriage.

HERB: We never fought per se.

Another interesting point that surfaced in the follow-up was the spiraling nature of change. The moment Dorothy got her parents out of her life, she began to fill up her life with more than just her husband. One senses from the way Herb talked about his wife that this lifted a load from him. In the past he had absented himself from his wife not only because of the anorexia but also because he had become everything to her, and this was too much of a burden for him. As she became less needy he felt he could approach and appreciate her more. This is an example of the spiraling of change, the husband responding to the wife's change with more change.

Living a Workable Reality

There was a tremendous need for this couple to say, "Whatever was wrong with Dorothy, it never affected our basic tie, the fact that we cared for each other." I sensed some exaggeration here, but this was fine. It was part of the renewal, this complementing of each other and building on what remained.

DR. FISHMAN: You used to say that you thought Herb was very critical of you, especially in public. Do you still think he is?

DOROTHY: No, not at all. Definitely. He's my biggest supporter. And he will say nice things about me in front of other people. A lot of that, you have to understand, was the way I was looking at things. You know, I wasn't looking at things very clearly. I made up an awful lot of things in my head. Oh, I believe that the situation was that way, but I turned it around so that I was the one that was put upon, I was the one that everyone was picking on. I could take any situation and turn it into criticism of myself, because I hated myself so much.

Dorothy is still focusing on herself to explain the events of the situation. She still prefers to say, "It was not that my husband was so critical—it was the fact that I was so sick that prevented me from turning things around." There is a beautiful consistency here in the self-sacrificial stance that she takes towards her illness and that now prevails. Of course, the couple has crossed a certain threshold; Dorothy is well, and even she realizes that there are limits to her self-sacrificing reappraisal of events. But the overall contour, the profile of the system, remains the same. Dorothy remains at the center, willing to absorb much of the blame, and in so doing bails out her husband. This pattern is of course reminiscent of the one that needed changing. But we must keep in mind that the system has in fact been rearranged. These people have been transformed and their problem overcome. The echoing of old patterns is merely evidence of the fact that a system can change radically and yet certain aspects return to a comfortable status quo.

However contradictory it might seem, this couple's return to a status quo is no reason for alarm. A neophyte therapist, upon seeing this kind of display, might believe that the structural patterns had not really changed at all, thereby confusing the general features of structure with the depth and rigidity of the patterns that had made Dorothy ill. The fact is that this couple was not behaving the same. If her husband were to stop being considerate, Dorothy might threaten to leave him and actually carry out the threat. What Dorothy did was shape a reality that did not challenge the present happy status quo. It may be that this was just one more method of conflict avoidance. But, on the other hand, when Dorothy talked about how happy she was and the fact that she was not symptomatic in any way, what she was giving us was, like all histories, a partial one, a story supporting the present status quo. At least in part, she was editing and restoring the image of how she believed a couple should be.

DR. FISHMAN: Do you feel that Herb and Greg gang up against you?

DOROTHY: Oh, it was bad. I would make it into a situation where the two of them were in cahoots all the time to check on me. You know, it wasn't like that at all. I saw it that way. I think the situation was that the two of them were concerned that my health kept going downhill, and I made that into criticism. I took that concern and turned it into criticism. Now he can't be in cahoots, because Herb and I are in cahoots with one another. So if he doesn't like it, we can tell him, "You're odd man out."

Here we see the limits of what change can bring about. The mother's account is fairly consistent with the pre-morbid phase of her pathological development. In the premorbid we saw an excessive tendency for Dorothy to overburden herself, absorb pain, and safeguard others. Here she returns to that sacrificial stance. This stance, however, is not consistent with reality. Her husband and the children were in cahoots against her. She was not delusional. In fact, her behavior encouraged Herb to form a coalition with the kids. That reality is now edited out, and amnesia prevails in the areas of the most severe conflict. This amnesia is not simply in the service of the ego, it is amnesia in the service of maintaining a new family organization that makes her happy. And her new image of the family is of a good family with strong roots and a history that is not rancorous and filled with conflict.

The couple's new alignment and strength become evident when Dorothy describes how they deal with their son. "If he doesn't like it, we can tell him, 'You're odd man out.'" This is a new alliance, a closing of ranks with her husband. The youngster must accept his appropriate place in the family. This is a fundamental realignment of the hierarchy that has prevailed in this system and represents a return to a more satisfactory organization.

HERB: And I think basically Greg is a good kid. We don't really have any trouble with him at all—other than spouting off about something. But as far as getting into trouble, not studying, into drugs, alcohol, or things like that—we don't have any of that kind of stuff. So, I see no problem. If he wants to stay home another year, fine. But after that he's getting the hell out. Because that's—you know, by then he ought to be able to . . .

DR. FISHMAN: Will that be all right with Dorothy?

HERB: Oh, yes.

DOROTHY: He has a part time job. Oh, it's just fine.

HERB: But maybe I'll have to pay for it. Get him on a campus where everything is closed in and I don't have to pay for a car; that's worth about five grand a year. But there's only one thing I'd like to bring up about this whole thing. When we came here—do you mind a little criticism?

DR. FISHMAN:　No.

HERB:　I don't think you were forceful enough in getting Dorothy to change her ways.

(*Dorothy laughs.*)

HERB:　It took a couple of bangs from her problems for her to finally wake up. Now, is this the culmination of the therapy that caused her to change her mind, or . . . ?

DR. FISHMAN:　After the therapy there were a couple of bangs?

DOROTHY:　No.

HERB:　Like, remember the last electrolyte imbalance, where she went to the hospital?

DOROTHY:　It was during the therapy, though.

HERB:　Was it the culmination of therapy that made her realize this after that bang? What I thought was maybe if somebody had said, "God damn it, Dorothy, you've got to stop all this stuff. You've got to stop indulging, taking laxatives and all that stuff . . ."

DOROTHY (*to Dr. Fishman*):　That's what you used to try to get him to do. You used to say, "How can you be so patient, why don't you just tell her to knock it off?"

HERB:　Yeah, but you were going around saying, "You're picking on me," or, "You and Gregory are picking on me." I don't know—the only thing is I don't know what finally woke her up—whether it was the therapy or being scared from the bang or a combination of it all.

This is a most revealing segment because it touches on the phenomena of crediting change. When therapy is effective one hopes that the participants own and possess the change without giving outsiders too much credit for the transformation. This process helps to crystalize a sense of autonomy, a sense of steering one's own life. Here we had the husband openly criticizing the therapist because he felt the therapist did not create sufficient change in his wife. He went on to talk about how certain changes had to occur after they left the session and claimed that it was from these experiences that the legitimate and decisive change took place. Herb clearly was not aware that these external incidents occurred because of the deliberate imbalance that the therapist had created in previous sessions. The forces for change had been prepared in the therapy, forces that allowed Dorothy to attack her husband and allowed him to fight back and even threaten to leave. The conflict, disgust, and survival that took place outside the treatment room carried out sequences instigated by the therapy. In terms of the overall therapy these operations between husband and wife turned out to be especially powerful.

DR. FISHMAN: I think you contributed to waking Dorothy up. Because I kept saying, "You need to be there for your wife."

DOROTHY: But I can tell you another thing from my point of view. The last time I was in the hospital, Herb came to see me, and I've never seen him so completely disgusted with me. There was no sympathy at all. He said, "I am so sick of you. I'm sick of what you're doing, I can't take it any more." I really got scared I was going to lose him. I felt at that moment, here you are, eighty pounds, with your face twisted. I couldn't move my face any more, I mean it was just over to the side. My hands were like claws, and I thought, who would ever bed you? And I felt he was going to go. I think I got scared.

It was not merely insight that made her realize she was desperate and had to change direction. A new interactional template had been created in therapy that could then be generalized outside of therapy. In this case the new paradigm for behavior was the challenge, the direct confrontation and the ultimatum. Herb utilized this template to challenge his wife and say, "Listen, if you don't shape up, I'm going to leave."

HERB: I thought you were going, too, but not that way, not through the divorce court.

The key challenging reaction of the husband had been made possible by a variety of sequences engineered by the therapist. First the wife was supported and pushed to attack her husband, to get out all of her complaints against him. This process of attack was carried to such an extreme that the unbalancing event was finally allowed to happen. Feeling assaulted enough now to be able to make complaints, the husband then did all of *his* reacting. Herb's assertive move in not allowing himself to be manipulated by the power of the symptom, the anorexia, was an eventual result of previous sequences in which his wife had been allowed to gain ascendancy and to punish him. Without that kind of preparation he could never have done what turned out to be decisive in fostering his wife's change. After that key event in the hospital, Dorothy finally retreated from anorexia. She dropped the use of laxatives and placed herself on the road to physical and emotional recovery. In the next segment Dorothy was seen alone.

DR. FISHMAN: What is your weight now?

DOROTHY: My weight now is about one hundred fifteen, up from eighty.

DR. FISHMAN: And is that pretty stable?

DOROTHY: It's been that way for about a year I guess.

DR. FISHMAN: What are the positive parts of your life?

DOROTHY: You once asked me this and it's always stayed in my mind. You said to me, "What would you ever do to have fun?" At that time we sat—I must have been in here twenty minutes, I couldn't think of one thing to do in my life that would be fun. Not one thing! Now I can think of a million things that are fun.

DR. FISHMAN: Like what?

DOROTHY: Staying up all night and watching cable TV movies and drinking orange soda. I mean, that's fun!

DR. FISHMAN: Alone or with Herb?

DOROTHY: Alone, or with Herb, whatever. Going on vacations is fun. Snorkeling is fun. Playing is fun.

DR. FISHMAN: Do you take vacations together?

DOROTHY: Yes. Just going out on a Saturday and going to New York or looking in stores or something like that—that's fun. Almost anything is fun now. In fact it's hard to find a bummer now.

DR. FISHMAN: Do you think Herb feels the same way?

DOROTHY: Oh, yes, I really think so. I think that he feels that life is a lot happier.

DR. FISHMAN: What have you learned? What would you do differently since you got better?

DOROTHY: Oh, well, of course I don't think I ever would have let myself get in that predicament in the first place. I think in retrospect, fifteen years ago I should have come for therapy. If I had come fifteen years ago, I would have been a different person a lot sooner. And that's where I made my mistake. Therapy was the *last* resort for me. It should have been the first resort. And that's why now I don't mind telling anybody. If you have a problem, that's the thing to do.

Fighting Entropy

When there is change the participants frequently have to fight against the system's natural tendency toward disorganization. Dorothy and her family had to maintain a constant exertion toward change to prevent the previous disorganization from returning. Any detailed examination during follow-up involves identifying the homeostatic forces that the people are now resisting and attempting to change. It is only realistic that those forces will not go away easily; they tend to reassert themselves. A good example is presented by Dorothy in the next sequence. She explains how her parents fight for the position to be benevolent, to be active and influential in her life. The parents' efforts to remain indispensable to her are irresistible, and the price of this woman's freedom is eternal vigilance.

DR. FISHMAN: What else have you learned in terms of your behavior? You mentioned to me at one point that you learned to stay out of your parents' marriage. Do you still feel that strongly?

DOROTHY: Oh, yes. I'll just give you an example. The day it snowed, Thursday, my mother called me on the phone and said, "Are you going on vacation this year?" And I have been telling her, "Oh, I don't know whether we're going this winter, the kids are in school, everything costs so much." Well, in the back of my mind I know very well we're going to go somewhere in March. When she called me up Thursday, she said, "Oh, well, I'll give you one thousand dollars." I said, "Why do you have to give me one thousand dollars?" She said, "So you can go on vacation with Herb." I said, "I don't want that one thousand dollars. Take that one thousand dollars and go on vacation yourself." "No," she says. "We don't need it. You bring sunshine into our lives, and you're always so cheerful." And I thought to myself, once again, I'm the only reason those two people exist. And it's the truth. But I have to work to stay out of the center of their existence, to make something else the center. And that's when I retreat. As long as I can keep her with her friends. I keep saying, "Make sure you keep your friends, you're going to need them. Your friends are so wonderful." Some of them are old hags— they're the worst gossiping biddies—but as long as she has them, they're something she can be interested in. So I have to stay out of that center and I know how to do that now. I know how to pull back now.

That the participants can tolerate and forgive some of one another's worst features is an indication that systems can change radically and still retain some quality of interdependence.

DOROTHY: But I don't feel guilty about it anymore. Another thing I learned was that it was okay that they were human and they made mistakes. And I think I learned not to hate. They can make their mistakes, that's fine. I don't have that same feeling of hatred anymore, or that frustration.

The changed system has allowed Dorothy to differentiate and mature. The capacity to forgive the parent and not expect them to be perfect is an important change. It indicates that Dorothy does not hold them accountable for her problems and that the rigidity and striving for perfection that characterize a psychosomatic system are no longer present.

From Structural Change Freedom Emerges

DOROTHY: Whatever they did, they did for their reasons and it's okay because I'm okay and I have a choice now. I have a choice of how I'm going to live my life. I never felt that before—I never felt that I could actually *pick* what I was doing. Because there was always that nagging guilt that brought me back there.

DR. FISHMAN: You feel you're pretty much in control then?

DOROTHY: Absolutely. I can choose to do exactly what I want to do.

The desired outcome of therapy is an increase in the range of freedom for the participants in the system. It is not simply a lessening of the constraints imposed by the system but also an opening up of new contexts and new possibilities for behavior. Dorothy now had a sense that she could exist outside as well as within the system. And since the system itself was no longer so suffocating, she felt free both to maneuver within it and to get out of it when she had to.

Our aim as family therapists is to construct a language of freedom within complementarity, freedom within systemic stress. Perhaps the real goal of therapy is to create a system that the participants can exist satisfactorily within as well as get out of when necessary—in other words, to provide as much choice as possible. The therapist must therefore check for change in terms of choice. The participants should be telling us that they feel less shackled, more open to possibilities.

DR. FISHMAN: Why do you think now you can tell your parents to go away? What's different? Do you have any idea?

DOROTHY: It's like saying, which came first, the chicken or the egg? Because I feel better about myself now. I mean, I have a healthy body, I know it's strong. I think my self-image improved.

DR. FISHMAN: Do you think it has to do with change in your marriage at all?

DOROTHY: That's hard for me to say. I really can't answer that question, because a lot of it I will attribute to—you know, when you don't eat anything for a long period of time, you get awfully funny in your head. You really do. I mean, my nerves were just—I cried all the time. I was miserable. Sure my marriage changed, but it was very hard to relate to somebody like me. I was always cheerful and pleasant on the outside, but I spent an awful lot of time crying and being depressed. And you can't relate to a person that's in that situation. Herb really had his hands tied. He couldn't do anything because I wouldn't respond at all. Sure things have changed in our marriage, but I think the change came about because I got a little bit better and a little bit better and then I felt better about myself, pushed them [her parents] out, and then went more to him.

In a sense my question was a very difficult one. After all, how can the fish analyze the sea while swimming in it? The husband changed and became more considerate toward her; at the same time she drew the strength to throw the other, intrusive people out. Dorothy cannot say that the source of that strength was her marriage. What is evident to her, however, is that she was so consumed with fury toward her parents that she was not able to be there for her husband. She was hooked into the parental system, a daughter first and foremost. This changed when she changed her self-image, a process that began because of the husband's interventions. But that fact cannot be

*articulated. For Dorothy the change began with the arrival
of a new self-image. That, for her, was the initiating step.*

The Canary in the Mine

Coal miners used to take a canary into the mine with them. When
methane gas rose to a dangerous level, the canary would die, a sure sign
that the context was dangerous and evacuation necessary. In this family
Dorothy, in a sense, had her own canary: the symptomatology. When she
felt the symptoms coming on, she knew that things were not quite right.
She needed to locate the dysfunction—the poison gas—in her relationships with the significant people of her life.

DOROTHY: In the back of my mind, I'm always worried that if I do the
               least little thing, I'll slip back and I'll have anorexia again.
DR. FISHMAN: Has that happened at all?
DOROTHY: No. But I felt that I had to watch out in the beginning, had
               to be mindful of it. I said, *no, you're not going to do that.*
               There've been times when I was really tempted. Not so
               much now because the more I got out of the habit, the
               easier it got for me.
DR. FISHMAN: I would see those periods when you feel tempted to go
               back to the anorexia as the barometer that there are things
               in your life that are bad. If you pay attention to changing
               the things in your life, you won't go back. And you feel
               now that you have the power—I can see it in your family
               —that you all have the power to meet any challenges. If
               you meet the challenges—and life is always challenging
               —you won't go back.
DOROTHY: You mean, if you feel tempted, then look around? What's
               the situation in the family, what are the things that are
               making me unhappy?
DR. FISHMAN: Exactly.
DOROTHY: And that's what's making me go back to the anorexia.
DR. FISHMAN: It's a barometer.
DOROTHY: Is that what caused it in the first place?
DR. FISHMAN: We don't know what causes it, but we have an idea what
               changes it.
DOROTHY: Okay, that's the important thing. Who cares what causes
               it.

Summary

I learned a great deal from the follow-up with Dorothy and her family. Sometimes I wonder what would have happened if someone had worked with only the children individually. It is hard to imagine that their moroseness and their feelings of inadequacy could have been ameliorated without dealing with the deep problems in the family. In retrospect I think I would have worked differently with this family in regard to Greg and Jenny. I might have tracked them more closely to ascertain their developmental levels, through individual sessions with the two of them together as well as alone. If necessary I would have done more with them in relation to the larger context, even going so far as to bring in another child of their age to act as a co-therapist. Had I done this, Greg might have been further along in his relationships with peers, especially with girls.

Of course, in reality there is only so much one can do with a family without indulging in an interminable therapeutic process. Although I might have done more with the adolescents in this family, the results of the overall intervention were promising. As Greg and Jenny retired from their position as nursemaids to their mother they rapidly began connecting with peers, developing friendships, improving their school performance, and retreating from the moroseness that had characterized their personalities. These changes reassured me that there had indeed been a transformation of the system that directly affected these adolescents and significantly improved the quality of their lives.

12

Epilogue

How can the kids have hope when their parents don't?
—Mia, age sixteen

S I THINK ABOUT the adolescents described in these pages and the contexts in which they live I have a nagging feeling that something is missing from my analysis. Is the lens I have used too limited? In treating these youngsters I attempted to include all of the important individuals and agencies that appeared to impinge on the system and which therefore had to be involved in order to address the problem and produce change. But I have ignored the broader context: no picture of the forces impacting the adolescent is complete without considering the larger social context within which the child is maturing. And to a great extent this context is made up of profoundly disquieting social and political forces which affect our adolescents in varying degrees at different stages as they proceed to adulthood. Of course, our ability to deal with these forces in therapy is limited. But as the young girl quoted at the opening of this chapter says so poignantly, "How can the kids have hope when their parents don't?" Regardless of the enormity of the problems, we have a responsibility to try to do something about them.

What are some of the problems that stress our adolescents? Just picking up a newspaper one is struck by the amorality of our leaders. In a recent article in *Time* magazine on the state of American ethics, Ezra Bowen (1987) quoted church historian Martin E. Marty as seeing a "widespread sense of moral disarray" (p. 26). Further, political scientist Steven Salkever is quoted in the same article as saying that "there was a traditional language of public discourse, based partly on biblical sources, partly on republican sources. But that language has fallen into disuse, leaving American society with no moral lingua franca" (p. 26). The moral beliefs of our grandparents no longer seem to hold. There is a popular consensus that moral disarray is rife. Also reported in the *Time* article (p. 26) is a poll by Yankelovich Clancy Shulman which reveals that more than 90 percent of respondents agreed that moral values have fallen because parents fail to take responsibility for their children or to imbue in them decent moral standards. Seventy-six percent saw a lack of ethics in business as contributing to tumbling moral standards, and 74 percent decried the failure of political leaders to set a good example. How are adolescents to know right from wrong when there are no trustworthy role models?

Of course, the stress emanating from this confusion can only be compounded by the fact that for the first time in history humanity is threatened with the very real possibility of total destruction. More nuclear weapons are being built every day. Even excluding an act of madness, the possibility of inadvertent war or a holocaust produced by an accident at some domestic reactor creates stress.

Another recently emerging stress on adolescents is Acquired Immune Deficiency Syndrome (AIDS). For our youngsters, sexual experimentation has new significance. The sexual freedom of their parents is no longer an option. Indeed, it has been propounded that "the only safe sex is abstinence." How do adolescents explore their sexuality under these circumstances?

To this list of stressors can be added the fear of becoming a victim of crime as well as the growing awareness of the scope and seriousness of global problems such as environmental pollution and overpopulation. It may seem paradoxical to conclude a book on family therapy, a field whose central tenet is relativity, by condemning this very tenet. But the fact is that living in an era in which truth is relative does add stress to the adolescent's life.

David Brock (1987), in an article on Allan Bloom's *The Closing of the American Mind*, gives an overview of the author's discussion of the quandary that afflicts young people. Bloom refers to the writings of the nineteenth-century philosopher Friedrich Nietzsche, who held that science had killed man's capacity to believe in God but left no moral substitute for

God, and quotes a remark by Fedor Dostoyevsky that Nietzsche had much admired: "Without God, everything is permissible."

Bloom asserts that moral relativism is the dominant force in the American university—where the teachers and parents of today's adolescents were educated. As a result, openness is the only moral virtue worthy of respect. Bloom says "Everything else—what Immanuel Kant called the Good, the True, the Beautiful—is relative" (p. 10). Bloom, a professor at the University of Chicago, does not place all of the blame on our schools and universities. Indeed, he holds that, "country, religion, family, ideas of civilization, all the sentimental and historical forces that stood between cosmic infinity and the individual, providing some notion of a place within the whole, have been rationalized and lost their compelling force" (p. 12).

How does this moral crisis affect our adolescents? They may be living in a world where they do not know right from wrong. I believe it is important to be discriminating about just what this situation implies in terms of the adolescent's experience: it generates confusion, anxiety, and disquiet. My hypothesis is that such factors result in the adolescent having an experience of diminished control over the world in which he or she lives.

There is considerable research supporting the premise that a sense of control is an important element in the maintenance of health. Meredith Minkler, in her article "The Social Component of Health" (1986), reports on a number of research projects in which increased social supports led to improved health. She cites evidence from a study of seven thousand California residents who were followed over a nine-year period. The study found that subjects with few ties to other people had a mortality rate two to five times higher than those with more ties.

According to Minkler, other studies confirm that whether one looks at family relationships or at broader measures, there is a strong relationship between one's social support and one's health. She suggests that a promising explanation for the salubrious effect of increased ties is the hypothesis that, "over time, people's perceived sense of support from others may lead them to a more generalized sense of control" (p. 34). Says Minkler, this global need to have control over one's destiny serves as a likely explanation for the finding that social support is critically linked to health.

This, of course, is a well-developed notion—that with more support there is a greater sense of control. The control comes from a derived strength, a feeling that there is confirmation from the people around us. Reality is confirmation by significant others. Thus, having an increased number of significant others gives greater confirmation to a person's view of reality. From a more coherent sense of reality follows a greater sense of control. The world is a safer place.

What does this mean for family therapists and parents? Our task is to create a context for our children in which they have a sense of control. With a greater sense of control the youngsters will have more hope. I believe that one way for parents to provide that context is to let their children see them attempting to make some changes—even if only miniscule dents—in our world's serious problems. There are many social actions that we can take that will give our children the sense that we are attempting to have some effect, some control, over the social difficulties that have befallen our world.

One modest project I have been involved in is a television program linking families in Philadelphia and Leningrad—a simulcast "space bridge" in which two families will exchange not only greetings but experiences of family life. For example, they will discuss developmental pressures such as parenting, adolescence, and being a teenager in today's world. The goal of this program is to help the people of the two countries see each other as similar—to erode the image of the other as "the enemy." It is this distortion that our leaders use to justify the enormous stockpiling of nuclear arms. The viewing audience in the Soviet Union will be 150 million; in the United States 85 percent of television stations will carry the show. The hope of our group is that as these families meet, citizens of both nations will come to identify the people of the other country as self, not enemy. They will thus spark a sense of control precisely in the area where adolescents reflect the same feeling of hopelessness as most adults do concerning the tensions between nations.

I believe that parents of adolescents must demonstrate to their children a passionate concern for the world and for the future. They—indeed, all adults who deal with children—must model for them an atmosphere of hope and control, a paradigm of acting apart from the system. Our initiatives to fight social problems speak to the thwarted idealism of today's adolescents. They replace nihilism and depression with a sense that we can take control, we can work to end the sources of stress in our lives. This, I believe, is an ethical imperative of our generation for the next generation.

The ultimate complement to systems theory conceptualization is taking a model that sees the individual human being not only as a well-joined, articulated member of a system but also, at times, as an individual who acts asystemically when the human spirit prevails. The individual can be a member of a context as well as the *creator* of a new context.

References

Anderson, B. J., Miller, J. P., Auslander, W. F., and Santiago, J. V. (1981). Family characteristics of diabetic adolescents: Relationship to metabolic control. *Diabetes Care, 4*, 586–594.

Aries, P. (1962). *Centuries of childhood: A social history of family life.* New York: Alfred A. Knopf.

Barter, J. T., Swaback, D. O., and Todd, D. (1968). Adolescent suicide attempts: A follow-up study of hospitalized patients. *Archives of General Psychiatry, 19*, 523–527.

Bateson, G. (1979). *Mind and nature.* New York: Dutton.

———, Jackson, D., Haley, J., and Weakland, J. (1956). Toward a theory of schizophrenia. *Behavioral Science, 1*(4), 201–227.

Bayh, B. (1973). In Committee on the Judiciary, U.S. Senate, *Runaway youth* (Hearings before the subcommittee to investigate juvenile delinquency). Washington, D.C.: Government Printing Office.

Blos, P. (1979). *The adolescent passage.* New York: International Universities Press.

Bowen, E. (1986, May 25). Looking to its roots. *Time*, pp. 26–29.

Brion-Meisels, S., and Selman, R. L. (1984). Early adolescent development of new interpersonal strategies: Understanding and intervention. *School Psychology Review, 13*, 278–291.

Brock, D. (1987, May 11). A philosopher hurls down the stinging moral gauntlet. *Insight Magazine of the Washington Times*, pp. 10–12.

Brown, C. (1965). *Manchild in the promised land.* New York: Signet.

Bruch, H. (1973). *Eating disorders: Obesity, anorexia nervosa, and the person within.* New York: Basic Books.

Carlson, G. A. (1981). The phenomenology of adolescent depression. *Adolescent Psychiatry, 9*, 411–421.

Carter, E. A., and McGoldrick, M. (1980). *The family life cycle: A framework for family therapy.* New York: Gardner Press.

Carroll, J. C. (1977). The intergenerational transmission of family violence: The long-term effects of aggressive behavior. *Aggressive Behavior, 3*, 289–299.

Cassoria, R. M. S. (1979). Suicidal behavior in adolescents. *Acta Siquiatrica y Psicologica, 25*(4), 288–295.

Chess, S., and Thomas, A. (1984). *Origins and evolution of behavior disorders: From infancy to early adult life.* New York: Brunner/Mazel.

Drake, D. C. (1987, February 22). The mystery of teenage suicide. *Philadelphia Inquirer,* 12–30, 35.

Durkheim, E. (1951). *Suicide.* New York: Free Press.

Dykeman, B. F. (1984). Adolescent suicide: Recognition and intervention. *College Student Journal, 18:* 364–368.

Durrell, L. (1958). *Balthazar: Book II of the Alexandria Quartet.* New York: Dutton.

Erikson, E. H. (1958). *Young man Luther: A study in psychoanalysis and history.* New York: Norton.

———. (1968). *Identity youth and crisis.* New York: Norton.

Farber, E. D., Kinast, C., McCoard, W. D., and Falkner, D. (1984). Violence in families of adolescent runaways. *Child Abuse and Neglect, 8,* 295–299.

Finkelhor, D. (1979). *Sexually victimized children.* New York: Free Press.

Fishman, H. C., Scott, S., and Betof, N. (1977). A hall of mirrors: A structural approach to the problems of the retarded. *Mental Retardation Journal, 15*(4), 24.

Garmezy, N. (1983). Stressors of childhood. In N. Garmezy and M. Rutter (Eds.), *Stress, coping and development in children* (pp. 43–84). New York: McGraw-Hill.

Gelles, R. J. (1974). *The violent home.* Beverly Hills: Sage.

———. (1980). Violence in the family: A review of research in the seventies, *Journal of Marriage and the Family, 42*(4), 873–885.

Glansdorf, P., and Prigogine, I. (1971). *Thermodynamic theory of structure, stability and fluctuations.* New York: Wiley.

Goldenberg, I., and Goldenberg, H. (1985). *Family therapy: An overview.* Monterey, CA: Brooks/Cole.

Goldner, V. (1981, April). *The Politics of Family Therapy.* Paper presented at the Philadelphia Child Guidance Clinic, Philadelphia, PA.

Goode, W. J. (1971). Force and violence in the family, *Journal of Marriage and the Family, 33,* 624–636.

Grotevant, H. D., and Cooper, C. R. (1985). Patterns of interaction in family relationships and the development of identity exploration in adolescence. *Child Development, 56,* 415–428.

Hall, G. S. (1904). *Adolescence.* New York: Appleton.

Hampden-Turner, C. (1982). *Maps of the mind.* New York: Macmillan.

Hauser, S. T., Vieyra, M. A. B., Jacobson, A. M., and Wertlieb, D. (1985). Vulnerability and resilience in adolescence: Views from the family. *Journal of Early Adolescence, 5*(1), 81–100.

Henggeler, S. W., Rodick, J. D., Borduin, C. M., Hanson, C. L., Watson, S. M., and Urey, J. R. (1986). Multisystemic treatment of juvenile offenders: Effects on adolescent behavior and family interaction. *Developmental Psychology, 26*(1), 132–141.

Hogan, M. J., Buehler, C., and Robinson, B. (1983). Single parenting: Transitioning alone. In H. I. McCubbin and C. R. Figley (Eds.), *Stress and the family: Vol. 1. Coping with normative transitions* (pp. 116–132). New York: Brunner/Mazel.

Holmes, T., and Rahe, R. (1967). The Social Readjustment Rating Scale. *Journal of Psychosomatic Research, 11,* 213–218.

Howard, J. (1978). *Families.* New York: Simon and Schuster.

Jaffe, P., Wolfe, D., Wilson, S., and Zak, L. (1986). Similarities in behavioral and social maladjustment among child victims and witnesses to family violence. *American Journal of Orthopsychiatry, 56*(1), 142–146.

Justice, B., and Duncan, D. F. (1976). Running away: An epidemic problem of adolescence. *Adolescence, 11*(43), 365–371.

Kagan, J. (1984). *The nature of the child.* New York: Basic Books.

Keeney, B. P. (1983). *Aesthetics of change.* New York: Guilford.

Koski, M.-L. (1969). The coping process in childhood diabetes. *Acta Paediatrica Scandinavica,* (Suppl. 198), 199–214.

———. (1976). A psychosomatic follow-up. *Acta Paedopsychiatrica, 42,* 22–25.

Lappin, J., and Covelman, K. W. (1985). Adolescent runaways: A structural family therapy perspective. In M. P. Mirkin and S. L. Koman (Eds.), *Handbook of adolescents and family therapy* (pp. 343–362). New York: Gardner.

Levinson, D. J., et al. (1978). *Seasons of a man's life.* New York: Ballantine.

Lieberman, R. P., Cardin, V., Gill, C. W., Falloon, I., and Evans, C. D. (1987). Behavioral family management of schizophrenia: clinical outcome and costs. *Psychiatric Annals, 17*(9), 610–619.

Mackay, A. (1977). *Harvest of a quiet eye.* England: Bristol Institute of Physics.

Mattsson, A., Seese, L. R., and Hawkins, J. W. (1969). Suicidal behavior as a child psychiatric emergency. *Archives of General Psychiatry, 20,* 100–109.

McKenry, P. C., Tishler, C. L., and Kelley, C. (1982). Adolescent suicide: A comparison of attempters and nonattempters in an emergency room population. *Clinical Pediatrics, 21,* 266–270.

Minkler, M. (1986). The social component of health. *American Journal of Health Promotion. 1*(2), 33–38.

Minuchin, S. (1984). *Family kaleidoscope.* Cambridge, MA: Harvard University Press.

Minuchin, S., and Fishman, H. C. (1981). *Family therapy techniques.* Cambridge, MA: Harvard University Press.

Minuchin, S., Montalvo, B., Guerney, B. G., Rosman, B. L., and Schumer, F. (1967). *Families of the Slums: An exploration of their structure and treatment.* New York: Basic Books.

Minuchin, S., Rosman, B. L., and Baker, L. (1978). *Psychosomatic families: Anorexia nervosa in context.* Cambridge, MA: Harvard University Press.

Mrazek, D., and Mrazek, P. (1985). Child maltreatment. In M. Rutter and L. Hersov (Eds.), *Child and adolescent psychiatry* (pp. 679–697). London: Blackwell.

Neill, J. R., and Kniskern, D. P. (Eds.). (1982). *From psyche to system: The evolving therapy of Carl Whitaker.* New York: Guilford.

O'Brien, J. E. (1971). Violence in divorce prone families. *Journal of Marriage and the Family, 33*(4), 692–698.

Offer, D., and Offer, J. (1975). *From teenage to young manhood.* New York: Basic Books.

Petzel, S. V., and Riddle, M. (1981). Adolescent suicide: Psychosocial and cognitive aspects. *Adolescent Psychiatry, 9,* 343–398.

Rosenblatt, P. L. (1981). Youth suicide. *Editorial Research Reports, 1,* 431–448.

Roberts, A. R. (1982). Adolescent runaways in suburbia: A new typology. *Adolescence, 17*(66), 387–396.

Russell, D. E. H. (1983). The incidence and prevalence of intrafamilial and extrafamilial sexual abuse of female children. *Child Abuse and Neglect, 7,* 147–154.

Rutter, M. (1979). Protective factors in children's responses to stress and disadvantage. In M. W. Kent and J. E. Rolf (Eds.), *Primary prevention of psychopathology: Vol. 3. Social competence in children.* Hanover, NH: University Press of New England.

———. (1980). *Changing youth in a changing society.* Cambridge, MA: Harvard University Press.

Sabbatch, J. C. (1969). The suicidal adolescent: The expendable child. *Journal of American Academy of Child Psychiatry, 8,* 272–285.

———. (1971). The role of the parents in adolescent suicidal behavior. *Acta Paedopsychiatria, 38,* 211–220.

Scott, J. P. (1958). *Animal behavior.* Chicago: University of Chicago Press.

Sheehy, Gail. (1976). *Passages.* New York: Dutton.

Shostak, M. (1981). *Nisa: The life and words of a !Kung woman.* Cambridge, MA: Harvard University Press.

Steinberg, L. D., et al. (1982). Effects of working on adolescent development. *Adolescent Psychology, 18*, 385–395.

Stierlin, H. (1973). A family perspective on adolescent runaways. *Archives of General Psychiatry, 29*, 56–62.

Straus, M. A., Gelles, R. J., and Steinmetz, S. K. (1980). *Behind closed doors: Violence in the American family.* Garden City, NJ: Doubleday.

Teicher, J. D., and Jacobs, J. (1966). Adolescents who attempt suicide: Preliminary findings. *American Journal of Psychiatry, 122*, 1248–57.

Tishler, C. L., McKenry, P. C., and Morgan, K. C. (1981). Adolescent suicide attempts: Some significant factors. *Suicide and Life-Threatening Behavior, 11*(31), 86–92.

Trout, D. L. (1980). The role of social isolation in suicide. *Suicide and Life-Threatening Behavior, 10*(1), 10–23.

Varela, F. (1976). On observing natural systems. *Co-evolution Quarterly, 10*, 26–31.

Walkind, S., and Rutter, M. (1985). Separation, loss and family relationships. In M. Rutter and L. Hersov (Eds.), *Child and adolescent psychiatry* (pp. 34–57). London: Blackwell.

Williams, C., and Lyons, C. M. (1976). Family interaction and adolescent suicidal behavior: A preliminary investigation. *Australian and New Zealand Journal of Psychiatry, 10*, 243–252.

Yeats, W. B. (1928). *Among School Children.* In M. Mack, L. Dean, and W. Frost (Eds.), *Modern Poetry.* Englewood Cliffs, NJ: Prentice-Hall.

Young, R. L., Godfrey, W., Matthews, B., and Adams, G. R. (1983). Runaways: A review of negative consequences. *Family Relations, 32*, 275–281.

INDEX

Wertlieb, D., 200
Whitaker, C., 128, 240
Whitman, W., 6
Wife: accomodation of to husband in incestuous family, 142–44, 151, 153, 156; anorexia of, 16, 242, 255–56, 259–61, 269–70, 272, 278, 290–92, 296; in couples therapy, 242–97; defense of husband by, 96; efforts of at gaining authority over son undermined by husband, 20; exclusion of husband by, 147; fear of changes in husband after therapy, 107–8; responsibilities of in incestuous family, 139; separation from husband in incestuous situation, 152; *see also* Mother; Parent(s); Step-parent(s); Women
Wilde, O., 81

Williams, C., 160
Women: battered, shelters for, 82; in group therapy, 133, 136; sense of incompetence and, 130; sense of powerlessness and, 130; sexually abused, 127, 129; *see also* Daughter(s); Mother; Wife

Y

Yeats, W. B., 3
Young, R. L., 60

Z

Zen Buddhism, 161